# GOATS:
## Homoeopathic Remedies

# GOATS:

## Homoeopathic Remedies

by George Macleod
MRCVS, DVSM

Veterinary Member of the Faculty of Homoeopathy
Veterinary Consultant to Nelson & Co
Homoeopathic Pharmacy, London
Veterinary Consultant to the
British Homoeopathic Association
Veterinary Consultant to the
Homoeopathic Development Foundation

Index compiled by
Francesca Garwood-Gowers

SAFFRON WALDEN
THE C.W. DANIEL COMPANY LIMITED

First published in Great Britain by
The C.W. Daniel Company Limited
1 Church Path, Saffron Walden, Essex CB10 1JP, England

ISBN 0 85207 244 9

Production in association with
Book Production Consultants, Cambridge
Designed by Yew Design
Typeset by Anglia Photoset
Printed and bound by St Edmundsbury Press Ltd.,
Bury St. Edmunds, Suffolk
This book has been produced on part re-cycled paper

**Other works by George Macleod**

The Treatment of Horses by Homoeopathy
The Treatment of Cattle by Homoeopathy
A Veterinary Materia Medica
Dogs: Homoeopathic Remedies
Cats: Homoeopathic Remedies

# Contents

| | |
|---|---|
| *Preface* | xi |
| *Introduction* | xiii |
| The Nature of Homoeopathic Remedies | xiii |
| Potencies of Remedies | xv |
| Administration of Remedies | xv |
| Care of Remedies | xv |
| Nosodes and Oral Vaccines | xvi |
| Vaccination Procedure | xvi |
| Diseases of the Alimentary Tract | 1 |
| Diseases of the Respiratory System | 11 |
| Diseases of the Nervous System | 25 |
| Diseases of the Urinary System | 29 |
| Diseases of the Skin | 35 |
| Specific Skin Conditions | 39 |
| Mastitis | 45 |
| Metabolic Diseases | 51 |
| Specific Diseases | 61 |
| a. Diseases caused by Bacteria | 61 |
| b. Diseases caused by Viruses | 72 |
| Miscellaneous Specific Conditions | 79 |
| First Aid Remedies | 89 |
| Worming | 93 |
| Infertility and Irregularities of the Oestrus Cycle | 95 |
| Rearing of Young Kids | 105 |
| Materia Medica | 107 |
| *Index* | 161 |

# *Preface*

In compiling this outline of common conditions affecting the goat those diseases which are subject to control under the Diseases of Animals Acts & Orders have been deliberately omitted for obvious reasons. Also certain other specific diseases have been left out because they are not enzootic in the U.K. and therefore of limited interest to Goat Keepers in this country.

A section on Materia Medica has been included relating to remedies mentioned in the text which I hope will enable the reader new to Homoeopathy to grasp a little of the essentials of each remedy, its origins, range of action etc. These are summaries only. For a fuller description of remedies the reader should consult a standard Materia Medica.

Finally I would like to thank my secretary Mrs. Enid Abbott for giving up some of her leisure time to typing the manuscript and for persevering in the face of some rather unusual nomenclature.

# Introduction

This book has been written at the request of Goat Keepers who have asked for information on the homoeopathic approach to disease conditions affecting the species. It is by no means exhaustive and only the commoner remedies are mentioned in the text.

For readers who have little or no knowledge of homoeopathy a brief description of its essentials is necessary to the proper understanding of the role of the remedies in treatment.

Homoeopathy is a branch of medicine which states that any substance which can cause disease symptoms can also be used in the treatment of any condition showing similar symptoms. The principle of likeness between disease condition and remedy is thus emphasised. If we imagine the illness and the provings of the remedy to represent two clinical pictures we should endeavour as far as possible when treating the condition to match one picture against the other. The closer the approximation of the two pictures (the likeness) the more we are able to achieve satisfactory results. This is much easier to achieve in human than in veterinary medicine as subjective symptoms known only to the patient are difficult to elicit in animals. Mental symptoms are extremely important in treatment by homoeopathy in the human patient. Observation of an animal's behaviour and how it reacts to any given situation (including disease), to other animals or people, noise, climatic conditions etc. will in some measure compensate for the lack of communication by speech. In certain cases it may be possible to imagine how an animal is feeling, e.g. the one subjected to forced separation from others in the flock or those suffering postoperative psychological trauma. Fortunately the homoeopathic Materia Medica contains remedies which are helpful in these instances.

## THE NATURE OF HOMOEOPATHIC REMEDIES

Homoepathic remedies are derived from all natural sources, animal or biological, mineral or plant, and their preparation is an expert subject best left to a qualified pharmacist. Some ill-informed people believe that remedies are simple dilutions, but this is not the case. The attenuation, or small dose of the remedy, is dependent on the technique known as potentisation. Any substance can become a homoeopathic remedy, but it is of use only after the pharmacist has refined the crude product in order to develop its inherent properties, and render its medicinal energy available for use. Preparation of the remedy includes first dilution, and then succussion. The latter is essential to the procedure, and consists of a vigorous shaking by special equipment. Those dilutions prepared in this way are referred to as potencies, and are used in either of two ways: (1) the decimal system used largely in Germany and France, and expressed by the numerals/letters x and D and (2), the centesimal system favoured more in Britain and the U.S.A., and expressed by the letter c. They differ only in the degree of dilution and succussion carried out at each stage. The more we dilute and succuss the remedy, the more the energy is released, so that the curative properties of the drug are retained, while all poisonous or unpleasant side-effects of the crude drug are lost, e.g. the active principles of poisonous plants such as Aconitum Napellus or Atropa belladonna are rendered innocuous after the third centesimal potency. The power of the attenuated dose lies in its ability to permeate the cell membrane, and accepted laboratory techniques have produced proof of the activity of infinitesimal doses of homoeopathic remedies in potency. Without elaborating this further, we need only note that this use of the minute, or infinitesimal dose, is an essential corollary to the homoeopathic principle of 'let likes be cured by likes'.

Owners who are themselves homoeopaths will be acquainted with the 'sameness' of the remedies as regards their appearance and taste, but to others, to whom homoeopathy is new, I would draw attention to the following simple rules. The medicines all look the same and taste the same. It is important to realise that they are all different, and that one remedy cannot be substituted for another. Do not therefore remove any vials or powders from their boxes until they are required for use. As remedies are purchased with their name and potency labelled on the box, it is a good practice to write these again on the bottom of the box to prevent mistakes arising. The remedies should be kept in their boxes when not in use, and stored in a cool, dry atmosphere away from sunlight and strong-smelling substances such as camphor, creosote or carbolic. Do not, therefore, store the remedies in farm outhouses.

# POTENCIES OF REMEDIES

The potencies of the various remedies outlined in the text are offered as a general guide, and it may be found necessary according to the condition, not only to vary them or use a different strength, but also to extend the period of time over which they are given for longer than is suggested in the text.

Also, very acute conditions may require higher strengths of remedies than are generally outlined. I make it a general rule that the more acute the condition, the higher the potency needed, while chronic states involving tissue change are catered for by the lower potencies. This is not a hard and fast rule, as other practitioners of homoeopathic medicine have different views. This may appear confusing to newcomers, but the more they become familiar with the subject the easier it will be for them to arrive at the optimum potency for each remedy and condition.

# ADMINISTRATION OF REMEDIES

Remedies are marketed as medicinal tablets, granules (sometimes referred to as veterinary doses), powders, tinctures and dilutions in sterile water.

Generally speaking single animals should be dosed by allowing the remedy to dissolve on the tongue. It is not advisable to incorporate the remedy in the bulk food. Where large numbers of goats are involved the remedy can be dissolved in sterile water and then emptied inside the lips by means of a small syringe. Remedies can also be employed by injection, but while this method may appeal to those who consider that this is a more acceptable method because of its "conventional" appeal, it is not to be recommended. The reason for this is that remedies are absorbed through the mucous membranes of the mouth and thus gives the best results.

# CARE OF REMEDIES

The delicate nature of homoeopathic preparations renders them subject to contamination by strong-smelling substances, e.g. camphor, scents etc. and disinfectants; also by strong sunlight. It is essential therefore that they be kept away from such influences and stored in a cool dry place away from light. The use of amber glass bottles is helpful in this connection for storage of tablets.

# NOSODES AND ORAL VACCINES

For the reader who is new to homoeopathy, it will be necessary to define the terms 'nosode' and 'oral vaccine', and explain fully the difference between them and conventional vaccines, which are administered by injection.

A nosode is a disease product obtained from any affected part of the system in a case of illness, frequently fropm lymph nodes or from respiratory secretions, e.g. nasal discharges in a case of catarrhal fever, and thereafter potentised. In specific, i.e. bacterial, viral or protozoal disease the causative organism may or may not be present and the efficacy of the nosode in no way depends on the organism being present. The response of the tissues to invasion by bacteria or other antigens results in the formation of substances which are in effect the basis of the nosode.

An oral vaccine is prepared from the actual organism which is associated with the disease in question, and may derive from filtrates containing only the exotoxins of the bacteria, or from emulsions containing both bacteria and their toxins. These filtrates and emulsions are then potentised and become oral vaccines. Nowadays it is the custom to use the terms 'nosodes and 'oral vaccines' synonymously.

# VACCINATION PROCEDURE

In the context of homoeopathic medicine protection against specific disease is based on the use of nosodes or oral vaccines. Conventional vaccination relies on the administration of modified vaccines parenterally (subcutaneous or intramuscular) which, after a period of some days, produce antibodies against the disease.

In contrast to this method the homoeopathic approach is based on oral administration. The nosodes achieve protection by a total involvement of the defence system by a sequence which is roughly as follows: the nosode after being absorbed through the tongue activates the tonsillar tissue, regional lymph nodes of nasopharynx and mediastinum and finally the bone marrow and spleen. It will be appreciated therefore that eventually the entire defence or immune system is involved in the protective process. This is equivalent to natural infection, recovery from which brings a lasting immunity. The conventional method of vaccination by-passes much of the system described and consequently is a much less effective form of protection. Furthermore the persistence of an attenuated virus/ bacterium (protein material) in the system can lead to a state of low vitality with less resistance to other infections which may be encountered.

The vaccination procedure which the author adopts consists in giving one dose of the nosode night and morning for three days, followed by one per week for four weeks and thereafter one per month for six months. Individual animals in small flocks can be given the nosode direct on their tongues or dissolved in a little sterile water and drenched. Where large numbers are concerned the liquid nosode can be administered in feed, or sprayed over the muzzle by means of a spray gun. This latter method is very effective and is used successfully when administering nosodes to large or dangerous animals.

# Diseases of the Alimentary Tract

## 1. STOMATITIS:
### Inflammation of the Mouth

This condition affects the mucous membranes of the oral cavity involving the gums and tongue.

### CLINICAL SIGNS
Redness, salivation and possibly ulceration of various areas occur. Ropy saliva may be seen drooling from the animal's mouth, accompanied in certain conditions by a smacking sound. Refusal to eat may be present in severe cases. Secondary infection of ulcerated areas may show the saliva to be contaminated by purulent material.

### TREATMENT
The following remedies should be considered:
**1. ACONITUM NAPELLUS**  This remedy should be used early if a rise in temperature accompanies the condition. A high potency should be used e.g. 1m and repeated hourly for three doses.
**2. MERCURIUS SOL**  One of the main indications for the use of this remedy is profuse salivation which is often slimy in nature. Ulceration is usually absent but redness along the margins of the gums is a prominent feature. Suggested potency 30c three times daily for seven days.
**3. BORAX**  Indications for this remedy include the formation of vesicles as well as inflammatory changes. These vesicles tend to coalesce and rupture leaving a raw surface particularly on the tongue and dental pad. Animals which need this remedy are usually afraid to descend from any height e.g. from a cattle float or other transporter. Suggested potency 6c three times daily for seven days.
**4. ACIDUM NITRICUM**  If the inflammatory condition extends to the margins of the lips where skin and

mucous membrane meet this remedy may give good results. There may be extensive ulceration present. A high potency may be needed e.g. 200c repeated daily for seven days.

**5. BELLADONNA**   When this remedy is indicated the mouth is dry and presents a red shiny appearance. Accompanying signs include dilated pupils, excitement and a full pulse. The skin feels hot. Suggested potency 1m repeated hourly for four doses.

# 2. RANULA

This term denotes a cyst-like swelling beneath the tongue. It is usually caused by obstruction of a salivary duct.

## CLINICAL SIGNS
A globular swelling appears under the tongue and is soft and diffluent to the touch.

## TREATMENT
This is not easy by medical means but the following remedies may prove useful:

**1. APIS MEL**   This remedy is indicated because of the oedematous nature of the condition. The patient is worse from heat and is usually thirstless. Suggested potency 6c giving one dose three times daily for ten days.

**2. MERCURIUS DULC**   If the condition is attended by excess salivation as is often the case then this remedy may be helpful. Suggested potency 30c twice daily for fourteen days.

# 3. PAROTITIS

This term denotes inflammation or swelling of the parotid salivary gland and may be confined to one side only or embrace both sides. It may arise from exposure to cold winds or be an accompaniment to mild infections.

## CLINICAL SIGNS
The gland becomes swollen and may be tender to the touch. If bilateral a rounded appearance is given to the face.

## TREATMENT

The following remedies should be considered:

**1. ACONITUM NAPELLUS** If it is thought that the condition has arisen from exposure to cold winds, this remedy will help. A high potency is preferable e.g. 1m repeated hourly for three doses.

**2. BELLADONNA** If the gland is hot with possible extension to the ears this remedy may prove useful. Accompanying signs might include high temperature, dilated pupils and a bounding pulse. Excitement may be an additional sign. Suggested potency 1m repeated hourly for four doses.

**3. PULSATILLA** This remedy is indicated in those cases showing right-side involvement. The mouth is dry with a whitish coating on the tongue. Thirst is absent and the animal is restless with frequent changes in behavioural pattern. Suggested potency 30c twice daily for ten days.

**4. BRYONIA** Hardness of the gland is a feature of this remedy while pressure on the area is not resented. Mucous membranes of the mouth are dry while stools are dry and crumbly. Suggested potency 30c twice daily for ten days.

**5. BARYTA CARB.** If the condition affects young kids or old animals this remedy may help. There is a tendency for neighbouring tonsillar tissue to become involved. Suggested potency 6c four times daily for five days.

**6. CALC. FLUOR.** If the gland presents a strong hard feeling involving associated lymph glands this remedy may give good results. Suggested potency 30c twice weekly for four weeks.

**7. PHYTOLACCA** This is a first class remedy for glandular involvement generally. The swelling extends to the throat which may on examination appear dark bluish-red causing difficulty in swallowing. It is probably more useful in acute cases. Suggested potency 30c twice daily for ten days.

**8. RHUS TOXICODENDRON** With this remedy the left parotid gland is usually affected. Small vesicles may appear on the skin surrounding the gland and the throat becomes red and inflamed. Lachrymation may be present. Suggested potency 1m giving one dose daily for ten days.

**9. PAROTIDINUM** The use of the nosode is always indicated along with or prior to the administration of the selected remedy. Suggested potency one dose daily for five days.

# 4. PHARYNGITIS

Inflammation of the throat may have its origin in exposure to cold winds and also to changes in food.

## CLINICAL SIGNS
Difficulty in swallowing is usually the first thing the owner notices. On examination there is tenderness over the area involved. The inflammatory process may extend to associated glands and the ears.

## TREATMENT
**1. ACONITUM**   Indicated in the early febrile stage. Suggested potency 10m giving one dose every hour for three doses.

**2. BELLADONNA**   This is a most important throat remedy where general signs such as dilated pupils and hot dry skin are present. The patient may be excitable. Suggested potency 1m giving one dose hourly for four doses.

**3. MERCURIUS CYANATUS**   A membranous deposit is often present in the throat when this remedy is indicated. There are accompanying signs of generalised toxaemia. Suggested potency 30c one dose three times daily for five days.

**4. AESCULUS**   On examination the veins of the throat appear swollen and distended. Signs of liver disturbance e.g. jaundice and clay-coloured stools may be present. Pressure over the abdomen is resented. Suggested potency 30c giving one dose three times daily for six days.

**5. LACHESIS**   This is another important throat remedy indicated when external examination reveals the area to be swollen and tender. Internal examination reveals a bluish colour with slight haemorrhage. Suggested potency 30c one dose three times daily for ten days.

**6. ALUMEN**   Lymphoid tissue around the tonsillar area becomes hardened accompanying a similar state involving the superficial lymph nodes elsewhere. Suggested potency 30c giving one dose twice daily for ten days.

**7. RHUS TOX.** Dark redness of the throat is present especially so on the left side. Vesicles on the tongue and gums may be present. Suggested potency 1m one dose daily for ten days.

# 5. GINGIVITIS

This term indicates inflammation of the gums and apart from specific diseases, the condition may appear in a non-specific form.

## CLINICAL SIGNS
The gums appear red and swollen, the area adjacent to the teeth being more severely affected than elsewhere. Salivation is usually present, while ulceration may or may not be a feature.

## TREATMENT
**1. MERC. SOL.** Simple inflammation showing excessive slimy saliva is usually helped by this remedy. There is a dirty look to the mouth and a nightly worsening of symptoms. Suggested potency 6c giving one dose three times daily for seven days.
**2. MERC. IOD. FLAV.** The yellow iodide of mercury will be of benefit in treating those cases showing right-sided involvement. Suggested potency 30c giving one dose three times daily for seven days.
**3. MERC. IOD. RUB.** The red iodide acts more on the left side of the mouth and gums. Suggested potency 30c one three times daily for seven days.
**4. BORAX** Ulceration is present when this remedy is indicated. Salivation is excessive and frequently accompanied by a smacking sound. There is disinclination to descend from high objects e.g. when unloading. Suggested potency 6c giving one dose twice daily for fourteen days.
**5. MERC. CORR.** Somewhat similar to the other mercuries but symptoms are much more severe. There may be accompanying mucous stools. Suggested potency 30c giving one dose twice daily for seven days.

# 6. ACUTE INDIGESTION

This is usually a disturbance of physiological function, no pathological changes taking place. Overeating is a frequent cause and this may relate to normal feed or to the animal having access to palatable foods such as grain or cake and eating too much of either. Damaged feeds may cause the condition.

## CLINICAL SIGNS

Acute indigestion may be accompanied by bloat. Simple cases show as lack of appetite with a slight increase in the rate of respiration. The faeces may be hard or watery depending on the nature of the food taken. Rumenal contractions are usually reduced when the dung is dry or increased when diarrhoea is present. Rumenal impaction produces a doughy feeling with reduced stomach movement. Severe overloading of the rumen may lead to toxaemia if treatment is not started early, recumbency, sluggish reflexes and a sub-normal temperature being present.

## TREATMENT

The following remedies may be needed:

**1. ABIES CANADENSIS**  This is a useful remedy when simple overeating is the cause. Abdominal flatulence arises. Suggested potency 30c three times daily for three days.

**2. CARBO VEG.**  Indicated when pronounced bloating is present accompanied by toxaemia and tendency to coma. Suggested potency 200c one every hour for four doses.

**3. COLCHICUM**  Too much green food precipitating the condition calls for this remedy when bloat is also present. The bowels are usually loose. Suggested potency 30c three times daily for four days..

**4. NUX VOM.**  Indicated when the condition arises from the ingestion of indigestible fodder. Constipation is invariably present. Suggested potency 1m three times daily for four days.

**5. LYCOPODIUM**  Mild cases of bloat may benefit from this remedy. The lower right hand side of the abdomen feels full due to sluggish liver activity. Suggested potency 200c daily five days.

# 7. ENTERITIS:
## Inflammation of Intestinal Tract

This condition may follow acute indigestion or be secondary to some specific trouble such as mastitis or metritis.

### CLINICAL SIGNS
Diarrhoea occurs with evidence of pain. The animal refuses food. Shreds of mucus may be present along with blood, accompanied by straining.

### TREATMENT
The following remedies may be needed according to overall symptoms:

**1. ACONITUM** Should be given early if possible. It will help combat shock and calm the patient. Suggested potency 1m one dose every hour for three doses.

**2. ARSENICUM ALBUM** Restlessness and a worsening of the condition towards midnight suggest this remedy. Stools may be blood-stained and have a foul odour. Suggested potency 1m three times daily for four days.

**3. COLOCYNTHIS** Indicated when the animal lies down and probably rolls in pain. Arching of the back is noticed. Suggested potency 1m one dose every hour for four doses.

**4. CROTON TIGLIUM** Stools are watery and forcibly expelled. Itching of the skin may accompany the condition. Suggested potency 30c three times daily for three days.

**5. MERC. CORR.** Indicated when the stools are dysenteric and full of mucus accompanied by much straining. The patient is worse during the night. Suggested potency 1m three times daily for four days.

**6. RHEUM** Indicated when stools are mushy and smell sour. They may be dark brown in colour rather than greenish. Suggested potency 200c one daily for five days.

# 8. PERITONITIS

Inflammation of the peritoneal covering of the digestive

tract is rarely primary, being a sequel to one or other acute conditions, such as septicaemia arising from mastitis, metritis or liver abscess.

## CLINICAL SIGNS
Lack of appetite accompanies a rise in temperature and pulse rate together with increased respiration. The back becomes arched and a painful grunt is heard on expiration. The peritoneal covering can be felt as a hard board-like structure on deep pressure over the sub-lumbar area.

## TREATMENT
**1. ACONITUM** Will relieve pain and anxiety and lessen the shock to the animal's system. Should be given as early as possible. Suggested dose 1m one dose every hour for three doses.

**2. BELLADONNA** The patient shows a high temperature, feels hot and the eyes are dilated. Head shaking may occur. Suggested potency 1m one every hour for three doses.

**3. BRYONIA** Tenderness over the abdomen is extreme but hard pressure brings relief. Suggested potency 30c three times daily for three days.

**4. CANTHARIS** Severe inflammatory involvement of the greater part of the peritoneum suggests this remedy. The stools are bloody. The condition usually arises as a sequel to cystitis or acute nephritis and possibly metritis. Suggested potency 1m one dose every hour for four doses.

**5. RHUS TOX.** Indicated when relief is evident on movement. There is redness of visible mucous membranes. Suggested potency 1m one every two hours for five doses.

**6. PYROGEN** This remedy should give relief when a high temperature alternates with a weak thready pulse or vice versa, especially if the condition is secondary to a septic state such as metritis. Suggested potency 1m one dose every hour for four doses and repeated the following day.

# 9. BLOAT

Acute swelling of the rumen is a form of indigestion which can arise suddenly when gas in the stomach is produced faster than it is eliminated. A chronic form may arise as a result of prolonged bad feeding or mild gastritis.

## CLINICAL SIGNS
A fullness or swelling, small at first, appears over the left sub-lumbar region. This swelling increases rapidly as the rumen fills with gas. The animal becomes increasingly distressed and anxious looking. Soon the swelling becomes hard and tense while difficulty in breathing may be severe. The bloat may be frothy in nature when salivation is common.

## TREATMENT
If discovered in time the following remedies may help:
**1. CARBO VEG.**   This is a suitable remedy for less severe cases. Suggested potency 200c one every hour for four doses.
**2. COLCHICUM**   More acute cases may respond to this remedy. There may be accompanying loose stool. Suggested potency 30c one every hour for four doses.
**3. LYCOPODIUM**   This remedy while helping reduce the amount of gas will also aid the digestive process and help restore normal digestive movements. Suggested potency 200c one twice daily for five days.
**4. ANTIMONIUM CRUDUM**   This is a useful remedy in frothy bloat which comes on quickly after eating rich grass etc. Suggested potency 30c three times daily for three days.
**5. APIS MEL.**   The amount of fluid generated in frothy bloat suggests that this remedy should be useful. Suggested potency 30c one dose every hour for five doses.

# 10. JAUNDICE

Jaundice is a symptom of liver dysfunction and not a disease *per se*. It leads to yellowish discolouration of visible mucous membranes. Remedies which may help the function of the liver providing organic disease is not present include the following:
**1. CHELIDONIUM**   With this remedy the yellow colour of mucous membranes and possibly eyes and abdominal skin is quite pronounced. There is an accompanying tenderness over the right shoulder area. Sug-

gested potency 30c giving one dose twice daily for seven days.

**2. LYCOPODIUM** More chronic cases showing indigestion and flatulence may well respond to this remedy. Stools are dry and shiny with occasionally mucous covering. Suggested potency 12c giving one dose three times daily for ten days.

**3. BERBERIS VULGARIS** This remedy is indicated if there is tenderness over the loin area, evidenced by the animal tending to sink down when pressure is applied over that area. The urine may be dark with occasional traces of blood. Suggested potency 30c giving one dose twice daily for fourteen days.

**4. CHIONANTHUS** The liver is usually enlarged and palpable when this remedy is indicated. Stools are clay or putty coloured. Suggested potency 6c giving one dose three times daily for fourteen days.

**5. PHOSPHORUS** This is a very useful remedy to aid liver function and is more suitable to the excitable or easily frightened animal. Superficial haemorrhages may appear on gums and around the udder in female goats. Suggested potency 30c giving one dose daily for fourteen days.

# Diseases of the Respiratory System

## 1. EPISTAXIS: Nose Bleed

This is less of a problem in goats than it is in some other species e.g. horses but is occasionally seen.

### CLINICAL SIGNS
The bleeding may be confined to one nostril only when it is usually associated with dead lesions: or it may be bilateral when generalised upset is present. The character of the blood may indicate venous or arterial haemorrhage and care must be taken to differentiate local bleeding from that arising from pulmonary involvement.

### TREATMENT
The following remedies may be needed to control the condition:
**1. ARNICA** This remedy should be given when haemorrhage results from local injury. Suggested potency 30c one dose every hour for four doses. If the injury can be traced back some time two doses of a higher potency e.g. 1m should be given 24 hours apart.
**2. BELLADONNA** If there is involvement of the central nervous system evidenced by excitement and dilated pupils this remedy should help. Suggested potency 1m every hour for four doses.
**3. MILLEFOLIUM** Haemorrhage of bright red blood may be controlled by this remedy as it has a good reputation in nasal bleeding. Suggested potency 200c one dose twice daily for three days.
**4. MELILOTUS** Haemorrhages which arise from the ingestion of mouldy clover will be aided by this particular remedy. There may be haemorrhages elsewhere in the body. Suggested potency 30c giving one dose three times daily for seven days.

**5. HAMAMELIS**   Venous haemorrhages call for this remedy, the blood being dark and the flow intermittent. Suggested potency 30c three times daily for two days.

**FOOTNOTE**   There are many other remedies which could be used if the remedies outlined prove unsatisfactory. These include ACONITUM 30c: CROTALUS 12c: FICUS RELIGIOSA 12c: VIPERA 1m and PHOSPHORUS 200c. Reference should be made to a Materia Medica to find the main indications for each.

# 2. CATARRHAL RHINITIS – CORYZA

This condition is an inflammation of the nasal passages and is invariably associated with infection of one kind or another. Specific rhinitis relates to infectious disease.

## CLINICAL SIGNS
There may be an initial rise in temperature more commonly seen in young kinds. Nasal mucous discharge accompanies lachrymation due to conjunctival inflammation. The discharge soon becomes muco–purulent and coughing takes place. The mucosa of the nasal passages becomes red and swollen, and this swelling may extend to the sub–maxillary glands.

## TREATMENT
The remedies outlined here relate only to simple uncomplicated cases. Coryza associated with specific disease and secondary to pneumonia or bronchitis will be looked at under these conditions.

**1. ACONITUM**   This is a preliminary remedy and should be given early in the febrile stage if possible. Suggested potency 1m one dose every hour for four doses.

**2. FERRUM PHOS.**   There is marked prostration associated with this remedy. It is especially suitable for catarrhal respiratory troubles. Suggested potency 12c one dose every two hours for four doses.

**3. ARSENICUM ALB.**   Indicated when lachrymation is severe and a chesty cough is occasionally heard worse as the evening draws on to midnight. Nasal discharge is acrid and tends to excoriate the skin. Suggested potency 1m one dose three times daily for four days.

**4. PULSATILLA** When the inside of the nose becomes encrusted with scales and there is purulent lachrymation. Suggested potency 30c three times daily for five days.

**5. MERC. CORR.** Disease of the nasal bones suggests the use of this remedy. Discharges contain blood and mucus and show a greenish tinge. Suggested potency 30c three times daily for five days.

**6. HYDRASTIS** Simple catarrhal discharge which has a cloudy or yellowish tinge is associated with this remedy. Suggested potency 30c three times daily for seven days.

**7. ALLIUM CEPA** Bland watery discharges early in the affection indicate this remedy. Lachrymation is pronounced and the eyes appear red. Suggested potency 6c one dose every hour for six doses.

**8. DULCAMARA** This remedy should be considered when the condition arises as a result of exposure to a fall in outside temperature after a warm day as frequently happens in late summer or early autumn. Suggested potency 200c one dose daily for seven days.


# 3. CHRONIC RHINITIS:
## Chronic Nasal Catarrh

This condition may be associated with a chronic pneumonia or pharyngitis and can accompany abscess formation due to specific organisms.

### CLINICAL SIGNS
Respiration becomes difficult due to a chronic thickening of the nasal mucosa. This is accompanied by a purulent discharge which becomes thickened. Throat glands become swollen leading to further difficulties in breathing.

### TREATMENT
The following remedies should be worth trying:
**1. KALI BICHROMICUM** Purulent yellow discharge of a tough stringy nature calls for this remedy. Suggested potency 30c one three times daily for seven days.

**2. HYDRASTIS** Bland free-flowing discharges are associated with this remedy. They are usually colourless. Suggested potency 6c one four times daily for two days.

**2. MERC. SOL.** Discharges are greenish and tinged

with blood. Caries of nasal bones may be present and the condition worsens during the night. Suggested potency 30c three times daily for five days.

**4. SILICEA**   The discharges associated with this remedy are thin and greyish. Thickening of the nasal bones occurs. Suggested potency 200c one dose three times per week for four weeks.


# 4. SINUSITIS

Acute inflammation of the sinuses is relatively uncommon but a chronic form may follow after dehorning.

### CLINICAL SIGNS
A suppurative condition sets in and progresses to a longer-lasting purulent sinusitis. Proliferation of the sinus lining may accompany a necrosis of the bone in severe cases. Head shaking occurs and there is a rise in temperature in the initial stages. Purulent discharge from the nose is seen early but this may be absent later.

### TREATMENT
**1. FERRUM PHOS.**   Useful in the early febrile stage when its use may help limit the progress of the trouble to the purulent stage. Suggested potency 30c one every hour for four doses.

**2. HEPAR SULPH.**   Employed in a low potency e.g. 6c this remedy may help eliminate the purulent material from the sinus. The area over the sinuses is tender and painful.

**3. SILICEA**   Proliferation and thickening of the sinus lining leading to expression of a thin pus suggests this remedy in 200c potency giving one dose three times per week for four weeks.

**4. MERC. SOL.**   Purulent discharge from the sinus is greenish and tinged with blood. Suggested potency 30c one three times daily for five days.

**5. KALI BICHROM.**   When the pus is retained in the sinus and tends to become dry leading to expression of tough stringy mucus with a yellow colour. Suggested potency 30c one three times daily for seven days.

# 5. LARYNGITIS

Inflammation of the laryngeal area is frequently associated with other respiratory conditions such as bronchitis and pneumonia. It may be acute or chronic.

## CLINICAL SIGNS
Lack of appetite is an early sign and in does a fall in milk yield. A dry painful cough accompanies the condition which may extend down the respiratory tract. The chronic stage leads to narrowing of the laryngeal opening and produces difficulty in inspiration.

## TREATMENT
**1. ACONITUM**  Should be given as early as possible in the acute stage. Suggested potency 1m one dose every hour for three doses.

**2. SPONGIA**  This is a useful remedy for controlling laryngeal cough. The laryngeal area is sensitive to touch, and the cough is worse on breathing in. Eating or drinking ameliorates the cough. Suggested potency 6c three times daily for seven days.

**3. MERC. CYAN.**  If there is an accompanying membranous deposit on the throat this remedy may help. The patient may be feverish with dark red mucous membranes of the mouth. Suggested potency 30c twice daily for five days.

**4. SANGUINARIA**  This is a useful remedy for controlling any laryngeal oedema, which is often present. Suggested potency 6c three times daily for seven days.

**5. PHYTOLACCA**  Bluish red inflammation of the throat extending from the pharynx may benefit from this remedy. Mucus tends to gather in the region of the tonsils. The inflammation may extend to the parotid area giving the throat a swollen look. Suggested potency 30c three times daily for seven days.

**6. LACHESIS**  Severe swelling of the laryngeal area with a dark bluish purple appearance suggests this remedy. The area is painful to the touch. Suggested potency 12c one dose three times daily for seven days.

# 6. TRACHEITIS

Inflammation of the windpipe may be either acute or chronic. Predisposing factors include damp or unhygienic buildings leading to the establishment of differing infections. Dusty poorly ventilated buildings also play a part.

## CLINICAL SIGNS

There is an initial rise in temperature. Respirations become increased and there is a frequent dry cough which later may become moist. The cough is easily produced by pressure on the windpipe. Th.e chronic form may lead to the establishment of more serious trouble such as bronchitis or pneumonia. A muco-purulent cough is the main symptom of the chronic form.

## TREATMENT

**1. ACONITUM**   As in other febrile states this remedy should be given early. Suggested potency 1m one dose every hour for three doses.

**2. BRYONIA**   This is a useful remedy for controlling the dry cough of the acute stage. Pressure on the area may relieve the cough whereas with other remedies the cough may be increased this way. Suggested potency 30c three times daily for five days.

**3. DULCAMARA**   When the condition arises as a result of exposure to damp especially in late summer or early autumn. Suggested potency 30c twice daily for ten days.

**4. DROSERA**   A spasmodic cough resembling that seen in whooping cough suggests this remedy. Copious mucus is usually present. Suggested potency 9c one dose three times daily for seven days.

# 7. CONGESTION OF LUNGS

This condition may arise from an increased blood supply when it is termed active, or passive when there is an interference with blood supply. Exposure to cold and damp is a predisposing cause as also is transportation over long distances. it may accompany diseased conditions such as hepatitis or severe mastitis.

## CLINICAL SIGNS

A rapid rise in temperature accompanies laboured breathing. Frothy saliva is present together with a grunting sound when breathing out. The severity of the laboured breathing depends on the amount of fluid present.

## TREATMENT

**1. FERRUM PHOS.** This is a most useful remedy for the initial febrile stage of this particular trouble. It will help prevent the onset of more serious complications. Suggested potency 30c one dose every hour for four doses.

**2. AMMONIUM CAUSTICUM** This remedy controls moist coughing which produces a harsh sound. Suggested potency 30c twice daily for five days.

**3. ANTIMONIUM TARTARICUM** This remedy will prove useful for pneumonic complications accompanied by plentiful mucus. Suggested potency 30c three times daily for five days.

**4. APIS MEL.** This remedy should help control the amount of oedema which develops. Suggested potency 6c three times daily for seven days.

**5. ANTIMONIUM ARSENICOSUM** This is a useful remedy when the congestion is worse on the left side. There is a tendency to recumbency and swelling of the brisket area. Suggested potency 30c one dose three times daily for seven days.

**6. AMMONIUM CARBONICUM** This remedy is more suited to right-sided congestion which is usually venous in origin. Suggested potency 30c one dose three times daily for seven days.

# 8. OEDEMA OF LUNGS

This comes about in congestive states when serum from the blood-vessels finds its way into the lungs. Any stress factor may produce this and it can also arise from anaphylactic reaction resulting from ingestion of foreign material e.g. vaccine or sera.

## CLINICAL SIGNS

Sudden onset is accompanied by severe difficulty in breathing. Frothy saliva is abundant. The head is held low and thin mucus may run from the mouth. Grunting is common and auscultation reveals the presence of fluid in excess.

*TREATMENT*

**1. AESCULUS**  This is a useful remedy when oedema arises as a result of passive congestion. Suggested potency 30c one three times daily for three days.

**2. AMMONIUM CAUSTICUM**  Indicated when there is an accompanying exhaustion or muscular weakness. Mucus is greatly increased. Suggested potency 30c one three times daily for four days.

**3. ANTIMONIUM TARTARICUM**  Indicated when there is threatened pneumonia with excess mucus, although little is coughed up. The breathing is easier if the animal lies on its right side. Suggested potency 12c one four times daily for three days.

**4. APIS MEL.**  This remedy should help reduce the amount of fluid and indirectly aid breathing. Suggested potency 30c one every hour for four doses.

**5. ANTIMONIUM ARSENICOSUM**  Indicated in those cases where examination reveals greater involvement in the left lung. Suggested potency 30c one dose every three hours for four doses.

**6. AMMONIUM CARBONICUM**  When the right side of the chest is more implicated this remedy may help. Suggested potency 200c one twice daily for four days.

# 9. HAEMORRHAGE FROM LUNGS

This is usually secondary to some serious condition which leads to erosion or rupture of blood-vessels e.g. abscess formation or the presence of a lung tumour.

*CLINICAL SIGNS*

The blood may be bright red and frothy accompanied by difficult breathing. The condition is frequently due to a chronic underlying broncho-pneumonia and is often preceded by a history of nose bleed.

*TREATMENT*

**1. ACONITUM**  This remedy should be given if the condition arises suddenly accompanied by symptoms of stress. Suggested potency 1m one dose every hour for four doses.

**2. ARNICA**  This remedy may be needed if there has been a history of some injury or other to the chest, also in some form of heart trouble. Suggested potency 30c one dose three times daily for three days.

**3. IPECACUANHA**  Indicated when there is an accompanying nose bleed along with lack of appetite. The slightest exertion produces coughing of bright red blood. Suggested potency 6c one dose every four hours for five doses.

**4. MELILOTUS**  There is muscular weakness present when this remedy is indicated. It is often associated with clover poisoning. Suggested potency 6x one dose every four hours for five doses.

**5. MILLEFOLIUM**  Indicated when there is excess bleeding from the nose associated with a chronic lung condition. Palpation is present and the blood is bright red. Suggested potency 6c three times daily for three days.

**6. PHOSPHORUS**  Indicated when a harsh dry cough produces a rusty blood-stained mucus: often associated with an underlying pneumonia. Suggested potency 200c one daily for seven days.

**7. FICUS RELIGIOSA**  This is another valuable remedy when coughing produces bright red blood. Haemorrhages from other orifices may be present. Suggested potency 6 one three times daily for three days.

# 10. PNEUMONIA

This condition may take various forms e.g. Broncho-pneumonia with patchy involvement of lung tissue; this form is usually sub-acute or chronic. An acute viral or Pasteurella pneumonia also occurs when the entire lung tissue may be involved. The condition may arise suddenly e.g. Pasteurellosis or be more insidious in onset. Exposure to damp and cold are predisposing causes as also are fatigue and transportation. Any change in routine likely to lead to this could be a triggering factor. Infectious agents responsible include viruses, pasteurella organisms and also corynebacteria.

## CLINICAL SIGNS
A rise in temperature accompanies coughing, depression

and lack of appetite. Respirations are greatly increased. Clear mucus appears on the nostrils but this soon gives way to a more purulent discharge. Grunting and mouth breathing are seen in severe cases. Percussion over the chest reveals dullness over the lower area while emphysema is present over the upper area. Auscultation reveals a variety of sounds according to the degree of involvement.

## TREATMENT

**1. FERRUM PHOS.** This is one of the main early remedies in febrile respiratory diseases and should be given as soon as possible. Suggested potency 30c one dose every hour for four doses.

**2. ANTIMONIUM TARTARICUM** Indicated in moist coughing with patchy distribution of lung lesions. Frothy saliva may be present. Suggested potency 200c one dose daily for five days.

**3. BERYLLIUM** Indicated when symptoms are more severe than the clinical findings would suggest. Slight movement brings on coughing. Suggested potency 30c three times daily for four days.

**4. BRYONIA** Indicated in those instances when the animal is disinclined to move. The animal prefers to lie down and any movement brings on distress. Harsh sounds are heard over the pleura. Suggested potency 30c three times daily for four days.

**5. DROSERA** Indicated when the cough takes a spasmodic form. This remedy has given good results in the young animal. Suggested potency 9c giving one dose four times daily for three days.

**6. LYCOPODIUM** Indicated when the condition is suspected of being secondary to digestive or liver disturbance. Breathing is laboured involving independent movement of the nostrils. Suggested potency 200c twice daily for three days.

**7. PHOSPHORUS** When there is extensive involvement or consolidation of lung tissue together with rust-coloured sputum. Suggested potency 1m one dose three times daily for four days.

**8. TUBERCULINUM AVIARE** Again young kids may respond well to this remedy. The upper portions of the lungs are more frequently involved than the lower. Suggested potency 200c one dose daily for five days.

# 11. SUPPURATIVE PNEUMONIA:
## Pulmonary Abscess

This condition is frequently part of a chronic pneumonia complicated by the presence of purulent foci secondary to mastitis, metritis or some other septic state giving rise to metastatic spread to the lungs.

### CLINICAL SIGNS
Persistent cough and loss of condition are evident. There is invariably haemorrhage from the lungs and a purulent nasal discharge.

### TREATMENT
Purulent pneumonia is extremely difficult to treat but the following remedies may provide a measure of relief:
1. **HEPAR SULPH.** This is a useful remedy for septic states in general. Suggested potency 200c one dose daily for ten days.
2. **SILICEA** Poorly nourished animals showing greyish purulent expectoration may improve on this remedy. It is more suited to the chronic case. Suggested potency 200c one dose three times per week for four weeks.
3. **CARBO VEG.** A useful remedy in cases of threatened collapse after neglected pneumonia. Suggested potency 200c one dose three times daily for three days.

# 12. PLEURISY

Inflammation of the pleural membranes is seldom seen as a primary condition being secondary to pneumonia or pericarditis while a chronic form may be associated with lung conditions such as abscess or necrotic infection of the liver.

### CLINICAL SIGNS
There is an initial rise in temperature accompanying signs of lung involvement e.g. harsh dry sounds on auscultation. Respirations are increased when the condition is secondary to pneumonia.

### TREATMENT
1. **BRYONIA** Indicated when the animal resents being

made to move. Recumbency on the affected side is a pronounced feature, while pressure over the area relieves any distress. Suggested potency 6c one dose every hour for five doses.

**2. KALI CARBONICUM**   Indicated when the signs of pain are worse on the right side. There is early morning aggravation when cough is worse. Suggested potency 200c one dose daily for five days.

**3. APIS MEL.**   This remedy may help dispel any excess fluid in the pleural cavity. Oedema of the brisket may be seen. Suggested potency 6c one dose four times daily for three days.

**4. ARSENICUM IOD.**   Chronic pleurisy may be relieved by this remedy. It is useful for cases which are slow to respond. Suggested potency 30c twice daily for ten days.

# 13. PULMONARY EMPHYSEMA

This is seen as a sequel to pneumonia, extensive interstitial changes taking place in the lung tissue. It also arises as a result of continual respiratory distress such as severe dyspnoea.

*CLINICAL SIGNS*
Severe difficuty in breathing is a constant sign and may be of such intensity for the animal to exhibit mouth breathing. Saliva, frothy in nature, is usually present and harsh sounds are heard on auscultation. Rapid grunting breathing is usual along with increased pulse rate.

*TREATMENT*
This is not an easy condition to treat but the following remedies may give some relief:

**1. AMMONIUM CARBONICUM**   Indicated when asthmatic-type coughing is made worse in warm conditions. Blood may be coughed up occasionally. Lung sounds are worse on the right side. Suggested potency 6c four times daily for five days.

**2. ANTIMONIUM ARSENICOSUM**   Excessive dyspnoea which sounds worse on the upper left chest. The animal prefers to remain standing. Suggested potency 6c one dose four times daily for five days.

**3. ARSENICUM ALBUM**   For restless animals which

show a desire for small quantities of water, drinking frequently. Symptoms become progressively worse as night approaches. Suggested potency 330c one three times daily for five days.

**4. DROSERA** For the milder case showing spasmodic coughing and upper laryngeal distress. Suggested potency 9c one three times daily for one week.

**5. BRYONIA** When the animal resents movement preferring to lie down and remain still. Pressure over the chest wall produces an amelioration of the symptoms. Suggested potency 30c one three times daily for ten days.

**6. LOBELIA INFLATA** The animal appears better for movement, but worse after eating. There are frequent bouts of short coughing. Suggested potency 30c one three times daily for ten days.

# Diseases of the Nervous System

## 1. MENINGITIS

This condition is invariably secondary to some bacterial or viral disease, but a primary form can occasionally occur. The commoner secondary form arises as a result of spread within the body from some generalised condition. It may take a purulent or haemorrhagic form, the former being associated with pyogenic infections e.g. joint ill in kids, metritis in does etc. Metallic poisonings e.g. lead or copper can lead to haemorrhagic meningitis.

### CLINICAL SIGNS
There is an early rise in temperature in most cases. Restlessness and head shaking are common which can go on to pressing the head against any suitable object. These symptoms may be followed by periods of depression. Muscular twitchings and spasms may appear, the favourite area being the neck region but they are also seen on the flank. Retraction of the head occurs.

### TREATMENT
**1. ACONITUM** The early feverish state calls for this remedy. It should be given in high potency e.g. 1m three doses one hour apart.
**2. BELLADONNA** Excitement with dilated pupils, hot skin and raised temperature suggest this remedy. Frequent head shaking is seen. Suggested potency 1m one dose every hour for four doses.
**3. CICUTA VIROSA** This remedy is indicated when twitching of neck muscles occurs. The head is usually drawn back or twisted to one side. Suggested potency 30c three times daily for seven days.
**4. ZINCUM MET.** Head shaking and rolling calls for this remedy when there is an accompanying paddling

movement of the feet. Suggested potency 30c twice daily for ten days.

**5. APIS MEL.** The acute form is sometimes associated with oedema of the meninges and this remedy should benefit such cases. Suggested potency 30c three times daily for ten days.

**6. PLUMBUM MET.** Severe cases compelling the animal to bang or press head against the wall indicate this remedy. Suggested potency 1m one dose every hour for five doses.

**7. MAGNESIUM PHOS.** Muscular twitchings and spasms may be helped by this remedy. The animal may be highly excitable. Suggested potency 200c three times daily for three days.

# 2. CEREBRAL OEDEMA

This condition occasionally accompanies brain disorders of ruminant animals. Encephalomalacia is the commonest cause but it can also arise as a result of brain injury.

*CLINICAL SIGNS*
Blindness is an early symptom followed by convulsions and muscle tremors along with stretching of neck and back. Muscle incoordination soon sets in and the animal may become recumbent with increased convulsions.

*TREATMENT*
**1. ARNICA** If injury is thought to be involved this remedy should be given as soon as possible. Suggested potency 30c three times daily for three days.

**2. APIS MEL.** Oedematous states in general call for this remedy and it should therefore be worth trying. Suggested potency 30c three times daily for five days.

**3. CICUTA VIROSA** Neck twitchings and stretching the head backwards indicate this remedy. Suggested potency 30c twice daily for ten days.

**4. STRAMONIUM** When there is a tendency to fall to the left side the use of this remedy may help. Suggested potency 200c daily for ten days.

**5. AGARICUS** When there is pronounced muscle incoordination and staggering this remedy should be considered. Suggested potency 1m daily for ten days.

**6. STRYCHNINUM** Indicated when stretching of neck and back is prominent (opisthotonus). Suggested potency 200c one daily for seven days.

# 3. ENCEPHALITIS

This term indicates inflammation of the brain and can occur as a sequel to bacterial or viral infection.

*CLINICAL SIGNS*
There is early rise in temperature dependent on invasion by the causal organism. The heart rate is increased and dullness and lack of appetite are noticeable. Excitement may be an early sign. Brain involvement is evident by bleating, head shaking and staring pupils. This may lead on to head pressing, convulsions and champing of jaws. Muscle tremors appear on limbs and face. Unsteadiness of gait is seen and may lead to paralysis.

*TREATMENT*
**1. ACONITUM** The early feverish state calls for this remedy. It wil help allay shock and anxiety. Suggested potency 1m every hour for four doses.
**2. BELLADONNA** Indicated when there are convulsions, excitement and head pressing. The pupils are dilated. Suggested potency 1m one dose every hour for five doses.
**3. CUPRUM MET.** Muscle tremors, cramps and rigidity may be helped by this remedy. Suggested potency 30c twice daily for seven days.
**4. PLUMBUM MET.** This metal like the previous one has proved useful in many cases. Head pressing is very noticeable along with loud bleating. Paralysis of limbs could also be a feature. Suggested potency 1m twice daily for ten days.
**5. HYOSCYAMUS** Frequent head shaking calls for this remedy. There is also a tendency to muscle twitching. Suggested potency 200c one dose daily for ten days.
**6. STRAMONIUM** Indicated in vertigo with a tendency to fall or stagger sideways, usually the left. Suggested potency 30c three times daily for five days.

# Diseases of the
# Urinary System

## 1. ACUTE NEPHRITIS

This condition is an inflammation of the substance of the kidney. It is rarely primary more often being a sequel to some septicaemic infection e.g. mastitis or metritis. Poisoning by chemical mineral and plant agents frequently leads to nephritis.

### CLINICAL SIGNS
An initial rise in temperature is followed by loss of appetite and possibly increased respirations. Tenderness over the region of the kidneys is evident on touch. Frequent urination of small amounts of highly coloured urine is attended with occasional difficulty in passing. The urine may contain blood, pus and mucus together with excess albumen.

### TREATMENT
1. **ACONITUM** This is an essential remedy in the early feverish stage. Suggested potency 1m one dose every hour for four doses.
2. **APIS MEL** The early acute stage is usually attended by oedematous infiltration of tissue and this remedy will prove useful in such circumstances. Suggested potency 30c three times daily for five days.
3. **ARSEN. ALB.** This remedy is indicated when there is scanty albuminous urine showing shreds of mucus. Thirst for small quantities of water with a late evening aggravation also suggests this remedy. Suggested potency 200c one dose daily for seven days.
4. **BERBERIS VULGARIS** Tenderness over the kidneys and sacral area accompanies frequent urination, the urine being cloudy and containing a reddish sediment. Suggested potency 200c one dose daily for seven days.

**5. TEREBINTHINA**   If the urine possesses a sweetish smell and is blood-stained or contains pure blood this remedy may prove helpful. It is frequently associated with acute infections. Suggested potency 200c one daily for seven days.

**6. UVA URSI**   The urine may contain bile and pus along with clotted blood and mucus. Suggested potency 6c one dose three times daily for ten days.

**7. EEL SERUM**   If anuria (scanty urination) is present this remedy will help promote a reasonable flow. Suggested potency 30c one every half hour for four doses.

**8. COPAIVA**   When the animal is seen to pass urine with difficulty the urine coming drop by drop and having a cloudy greenish colour. Suggested potency 30c twice daily for ten days.

# 2. PURULENT NEPHRITIS: Kidney Abscess

This condition usually accompanies any acute or chronic septic condition which results in metastatic spread to the kidney via the blood stream. This is sometimes seen in navel ill or septic mastitis.

## CLINICAL SIGNS
Emaciation is usually present but the most definitive sign is the presence of pus in the urine. Tenderness over the kidney area (right or left) is usually present.

## TREATMENT
This should be aimed at eliminating the basic septic condition and the following remedies may help achieve this.

**1. SILICEA**   This is a very useful remedy in long-standing sub-acute conditions. Suggested potency 200c three times per week for four weeks.

**2. PYROGEN**   If the septic condition is acute showing an alteration between pulse and temperature e.g. weak pulse and high temperature or vice versa, this remedy should be considered. Suggested potency 1m one dose every three hours for four doses.

**3. HEPAR SULPH**   Pain over the kidney area suggests that this remedy may be useful as conditions requiring it are extremely sensitive to touch on pressure. Suggested potency 1m one dose three times daily for three days.

# 3. PYELONEPHRITIS

This condition is probably more commonly encountered than the previous one although the state of the urine is somewhat similar. It is usually secondary to some specific infection and has been known to follow a difficult kidding.

## *CLINICAL SIGNS*
A muco-purulent discharge sometimes follows a difficult parturition and kidney infection has developed as a secondary condition. Symptoms of colic may be present evidenced by the animal kicking at the belly and stretching out the hind legs. Frequent straining accompanies the passage of blood-stained urine containing pus.

## *TREATMENT*
**1. BENZOICUM ACIDUM** Symptoms of cystitis accompanying a strong-smelling urine containing catarrhal deposits suggest this remedy. Suggested potency 30c three times daily for five days.
**2. HEPAR SULPH** Tenderness over the loins and resistance to pressure suggests this remedy. It is very useful in purulent conditions generally. It is particularly useful in the acute form. Suggested potency 200c twice daily for three days.
**3. MERCURIUS CORR.** Slimy blood-stained urine together with a slimy stool may respond well. Symptoms are worse during the night. Suggested potency 30c three times daily for seven days.
**4. SILICEA** A suitable remedy for the more chronic condition. Suggested potency 200c one dose three times per week for four weeks.
**5. COPAIVA** Difficulty in passing urine which comes in small drops and accompanied by a greenish colour with albumen casts may indicate this remedy. Suggested potency 30c twice daily for ten days.
**6. OCIMUM CANUM** This is a very useful kidney rem-edy when the urine contains a reddish deposit and is thick, purulent and blood-stained. The odour has been

described as musk-like. Suggested potency 30c twice daily for ten days.

**7. CHIMAPHILLA**  Another useful remedy which may be needed when the urine appears ropy and shows a heavy deposit on standing. Straining to pass urine is noticeable. It is valuable in both acute and chronic conditions. Suggested potency 6c three times daily for fourteen days.

# 4. CYSTITIS

This condition implies inflammation of the bladder and may be primary or secondary to some infection. Acute and chronic forms are recognised. The acute form is usually bacterial in origin while the chronic form is often associated with gravel or sand in the urine.

## CLINICAL SIGNS
Frequent urination is the commonest sign, the urine containing blood. There may be considerable difficulty in passing, arching of the back and signs of pain are evident such as kicking at the abdomen.

## TREATMENT
The following remedies may all help.

**1. CANTHARIS**  This is one of the main remedies in the acute form. Scanty amounts of bloody urine are passed with severe straining. Signs of abdominal pain are present. Suggested potency 1m one dose every two hours for four doses.

**2. CUBEBA**  Profuse muco-purulent urination accompanying the more chronic or less acute form may well respond to this remedy. Suggested potency 6c three times daily for ten days.

**3. CAUSTICUM**  This is a useful remedy to follow CANTHARIS and will help prevent development of the chronic state. It is well adapted to the older animal. Suggested potency 30c three times daily for seven days.

**4. COPAIVA**  Indicated in catarrhal cystitis. Urine is passed with difficulty and has a sweetish smell. The urine is highly mucoid and cloudy. Suggested potency 30c twice daily for ten days.

**5. COLOCYNTHIS**  Arching of the back and kicking at the abdomen suggest this remedy. Signs of severe pain are present. Suggested potency 1m one dose every hour for four doses.

# 5. BLADDER STONES: Urinary Calculi

This condition is not uncommon in the male goat. Calculi start off as sandy or gravelly masses which eventually coalesce and accumulate in the bladder. They may block the entrance to the urethra causing distress when attempting to pass urine. Straining becomes severe. The condition is more likely to be seen in goats which are fed a high concentrate diet.

## TREATMENT
Remedies which may help prevent the formation of sabulous or gravelly material include the following.

**1. LYCOPODIUM**   The provings of this remedy show large deposits of reddish sand in the urine so logically in potency it should be considered as a preventive. Suggested potency 1m giving one dose daily for fourteen days.

**2. BERBERIS VULGARIS**   Like the previous remedy this also will help prevent the development of sandy deposits. Pain over the loins is an indication for its use. Suggested potency 200c giving one dose three times per week for four weeks.

Remedies which may help disperse or break up the stones in the bladder include the following:

**1. THLASPI BURSA**   This remedy has a proven value in this condition and will be found useful in mild and chronic states. Suggested potency 6c one dose three times daily for fourteen days.

**2. HYDRANGEA**   This is a principal remedy and has been used successfully many times. Signs of pain are present over the left loin. The urine contains white spiky crystals and thick deposits. Abdominal pain is present along with increased thirst. Suggested potency 6c giving one dose three times daily for ten days.

**FOOTNOTE**   Male goats should have access to a plentiful supply of clean water which may help limit the development of the condition.

# Diseases of the Skin

There are various disorders or affections of the skin to which goats are susceptible like sheep and cattle. They vary in severity and importance and most are reasonably well suited to homoeopathic treatment.

Non-specific conditions include eczemas of different kinds and photosensitisation. Specific skin complaints include the various forms of mange, Ringworm, Goat Pox and warts.

## 1. ECZEMA

This is a general term which includes any disturbance affecting the skin. Different manifestations include dry scurfy skin, broken or ulcerated skin with raw weeping areas and those cases presented as acne-like eruptions.

### TREATMENT
Remedies to consider for these non-specific forms include the following:

**1. MORGAN** This bowel nosode should be given as a routine at the beginning of all skin treatments. Not only does it help allay inflammations but it paves the way for other selected remedies. Suggested potency 30c one dose daily for five days.

**2. SULPHUR** This is a useful remedy when inflammatory patches appear on hairless areas and also above the tail. Animals needing this remedy seek out cool places to lie. Suggested potency 30c one daily for ten days.

**3. ARSENICUM ALBUM** Indications for this remedy include a harsh dry coat with plentiful scurf and excessive itching. The animal shows thirst for small quantities of water. There may be an accompanying diarrhoea. Suggested potency 1m one dose daily for seven days.

**4. MERC. CORR.** This remedy should be considered when large raw weeping areas occur. These become secondarily infected when the areas become purulent. Loose mucous stools may accompany the condition. Suggested potency 30c twice daily for ten days.

**5. ECHINACEA** Indicated in cases showing extensive acne-like eruptions often dependent on an underlying inflammatory process. Suggested potency 6c one three times daily for seven days.

**6. HEPAR SULPH.** This remedy may be needed when the skin shows multiple abscess-like eruptions like boils especially when these are extremely sensitive to touch. Suggested potency 30c twice daily for ten days.

**7. GRAPHITES** If the skin lesions take the form of raw areas especially in the folds of the skin between the fore or hind legs and secreting a sticky discharge this remedy may help. Suggested potency 30c twice daily for ten days.

**FOOTNOTE** There are many other remedies which could be indicated depending on overall presentation of the condition. Reference should be made to a Materia Medica if in doubt about any particular one.

# 2. PHOTOSENSITISATION

This term implies a sensitivity to strong sunlight affecting unpigmented areas of the skin, and as such is more likely to be seen in breeds such as the Saanen, Norwegian Dairy and others.

The condition is frequently associated with the ingestion of certain plants particularly St. John's Wort (Hypericum) which appears to be a triggering factor.

### CLINICAL SIGNS
A dermatitis-like eruption first appears on the affected part which eventually becomes necrosed. Oozing of serum and swelling accompanying the dermatitis. Lesions may be seen around the eyes, muzzle, teats and along the back and shoulder areas. Internal derangement may be manifested by jaundice. If this appears there may be lachrymation, salivation and diarrhoea. Itching and head-shaking occur and the muzzle assumes a coppery appearance.

*TREATMENT*
**1. ARSENICUM ALBUM**  The use of this remedy will help reduce the irritation and promote the growth of new hair. Suggested potency 30c one dose twice daily for ten days.

**2. SULPHUR**  Any cases showing an accompanying redness and swelling may need this remedy. It will also aid the action of more selective remedies. Suggested potency 6c one dose three times daily for three days.

**3. RHUS TOXICODENDRON**  This remedy should help in the early acute stage associated with inflammation and oozing of serum. Suggested potency 1m one dose every three hours for four doses.

**4. CHELIDONIUM**  This is a useful remedy if jaundice is seen. It will tone up the liver and act constitutionally. Suggested potency 30c one three times daily for seven days.

**5. HYPERICUM**  This remedy should help relieve any pain associated with nerve endings in the skin which is frequently the case. Suggested potency 1m one dose daily for seven days.

# 3. FACIAL URTICARIA

Sometimes referred to as Blaine, this condition is allergic in origin probably from ingestion of certain plants and is manifested by oedematous swelling of facial tissues giving the animal a puffy bloated look. The eyelids are affected and lachrymation occurs.

*TREATMENT*
The main remedy to consider is *URTICA URENS* in 30c potency giving a dose every hour for four doses.

# 4. ABSCESSES

These may be either acute or chronic, specific (associated with certain diseases) or non-specific. They arise because of secondary infection from pus-yielding organisms such as Staphylococci or Streptococci. Acute abscess takes the form of a painful swelling when the animal resents touch while many chronic forms tend to coalesce and form fistulous tracts.

## TREATMENT

There are many good remedies which are indicated as follows:

**1. HEPAR SULPH.** This remedy has a dual function depending on the potency employed e.g. low potencies 6c–12c help the abscess to mature quickly while higher ones e.g. 200–1m tend to abort the suppurative process in the early stages. Needless to say if an abscess has reached a certain stage it will be better to hasten its maturation rather than attempt to suppress it.

**2. SILICEA** This is a very useful remedy in chronic abscess formation where fistulae tend to develop. Suggested potency 200c one three times per week for four weeks.

**3. TARENTULA CUBENSIS.** This remedy will be found useful if an abscess becomes hard with a purplish surround threatening necrosis of adjacent tissues. There is inflammation of underlying areas (Cellulitis) and pain can be severe. Suggested potency 30c three times daily for seven days.

**4. GUNPOWDER** This remedy has proved useful in the treatment of multiple small abscesses due to pyaemia. Suggested potency 6x one three times daily for seven days.

**5. STAPHYLOCOCCUS OR STREPTOCOCCUS NOSODE** These nosodes can be combined and given along with the selected remedy in a dosage of one daily of 30c potency for five days.

**FOOTNOTE** Externally a lotion of **HYPERCAL** (a mixture of Hypericum and Calendula) diluted 1/10 should be employed to clean out the abscess once it has opened. It can profitably be combined with a 1/3 dilution of Hydrogen Peroxide which will help aerate the area.

# Specific Skin Conditions

## 1. MANGE

This condition, also referred to as scabies or itch, is due to a mite which parasitizes the skin causing varying degrees of infestation. It is customary to recognise different types viz. Psoroptic, Sarcoptic, Demodectic and Chorioptic.

**A. PSOROPTIC MANGE** In the goat this type is much less severe than the corresponding condition in sheep (Sheep Scab) and is caused by a different species of mite. The owner's attention may first be drawn to the animal shaking its head as a predilection site is the ear. Spread may take place to the top of the head and down the neck to the shoulder area. The skin becomes dry and scurfy and itching may cause secondary superficial infection when purulent areas may appear.

**B. SARCOPTIC MANGE** This is a more severe type causing extensive skin lesions of a dry scurfy or scabby nature. Itching could be intense. If allowed to develop the skin eventually assumes a wrinkled leathery appearance. Young kids are equally susceptible.

**C. DEMODECTIC MANGE** This form is associated with involvement of hair follicles where the mites produce a pustular eruption leading to the formation of small abscesses. If undetected it can become extensive spreading from the neck to the front legs and shoulder, occasionally also on the head and around the eyes. Young animals are mainly affected but it is not contagious.

**D. CHORIOPTIC MANGE** This form is sometimes referred to as leg mange. The mites attack the skin of the lower limbs causing bare patches which are associated with itch and general irritation. The affected animal may be seen to stamp the feet or bite the infected areas.

## TREATMENT

The following remedies which apply to all forms of mange will greatly aid the action of external dressings or washes or dips. They are not intended as a substitute.

**1. SULPHUR**  This is a good general remedy which will produce a constitutional state unfavourable to the mites. Suggested potency 30c once daily for fourteen days.

**2. PSORINUM**  This nosode has been developed from the scabies vesicle and will help control the severe itching which attends particularly the sarcoptic form. Affected animals needing this remedy seek out warm places in which to lie. Suggested potency 30c one daily for ten days.

**3. KALI ARSENICUM**  A useful remedy for the sarcoptic form where the skin becomes thickened into leathery folds. Suggested potency 200c three times per week for four weeks.

**4. HEPAR SULPH.**  This remedy is more suitable for treatment of the Demodectic form. It will limit the development of pustules. Suggested potency 30c twice daily for ten days.

**5. GRAPHITES**  In the chorioptic form this remedy will probably be more suitable than some others. It will help to dry any lesion and prevent secondary infection. Suggested potency 30c twice daily for fourteen days.

**6. MALANDRINUM**  This nosode could also be used in the chorioptic form as it has proved beneficial in similar forms of skin complaints affecting the lower limbs. A potency of 200c should be given once per week for four weeks.


# 2. RINGWORM

This is a superficial fungal condition which can affect all age groups, quickly spreading to in-contact animals when they are housed together, in the winter months. Various species of fungi are associated with it, chief among them being one called Trichophyton verrucosum.

## CLINICAL SIGNS

The lesions assume a circular appearance and in severe cases may coalesce producing an extensive denuded area. The skin becomes dry and scaly but in contrast to the disease in cattle itching is usually absent.

## TREATMENT

Apart from topical applications the following remedies are worth considering in raising the animal's resistance to infection.

**1. BACILLINUM**   This nosode has proved extremely effective in many cases both in goats and cattle. Suggested potency 200c one per week for four weeks.

**2. TELLURIUM**   The ring or circular nature of the lesion suggests that this remedy could prove useful. It has a beneficial effect on the skin in general. Suggested potency 30c twice daily for ten days.

**3. KALI ARSENICUM**   The dry scurfy scab-like condition of the skin which develops should be helped by this remedy, and it will prevent the formation of leathery tissue. Suggested potency 200c three times per week for four weeks.

**4. TRICHOPHYTON NOSODE**   This can be combined with any selected remedy and given once daily for five days in a potency of 30c.

# 3.  GOAT POX

This is a vesicular and pustular condition characterised by eruptions on the skin of the udder and teats. it is invariably mild in character as seen in the U.K. A specific virus is responsible and the condition can be transmitted from one animal to another.

## CLINICAL SIGNS

Four distinct stages are recognised in the course of this condition viz. papular, vesicular, pustular and scab. The papular stage is commonly a small nodule which develops into the vesicular stage where fluid develops in the lesion; this leads on to the pustular stage when secondary infection contaminates the vesicular fluid; this eventually leads to the scab or healing stage. There may be an early transient fever but this could go unnoticed in very mild cases. The udder and teats are sensitive to the touch and lesions are normally confined to these areas. The period of time from the appearance of a papule to the healing scab stage is roughly eight days.

## TREATMENT

Although the condition is usually mild the use of one or other of the following remedies will cut short the infective process and prevent secondary infection of pustules which frequently occurs if the condition is allowed to run its course.

**1. ANTIMONIUM CRUDUM** This remedy is associated with typical papular and vescular skin lesions especially with a dry skin. Signs of indigestion may be present. Suggested potency 6c one three times daily for three days.

**2. CUPRUM ACETICUM** This is a leading remedy for pox-like eruptions accompanied by muscular stiffness and spasm. Loose bowels may accompany the condition. Suggested potency 6c one three times daily for four days.

**3. KALI BICHROMICUM** This remedy may be needed when the pustules assume a crater-like appearance with a yellowish base and discharge. Suggested potency 30c one twice daily for five days.

**4. RANUNCULUS BULBOSUS** This is another useful remedy for the vesicular stage especially if the lesions are more pronounced on the udder. Suggested potency 6c one three times daily for four days.

**5. VARIOLINUM** This nosode may be used either by itself or in conjunction with one or other of the above remedies. Suggested potency 30c one daily for five days.

**6. HYPERCAL LOTION** A dilution of 1/10 will considerably aid the healing of the pustular stage if applied locally once or twice daily.

**PREVENTION** A course of Variolinum 30c will be of benefit in controlling the condition. One dose per week for four weeks should be given to all in-contact animals and repeated once per month for three months.

# 4. WARTS ON TEATS

These are included under specific conditions as it is thought by some authorities that they are viral in origin. They are occasionally met with and are not usually serious. They are unsightly and prone to bleeding. They can be controlled by the use of one or other of the following remedies:

**1. CALCAREA CARBONICA** This is a useful

remedy for young does usually bleed. Suggested potency 30c one dose twice weekly for four weeks.

**2. CAUSTICUM** This remedy relates more to the older doe and is more likely to be needed to treat warts which have a cauliflower-like appearance. They tend to bleed easily if handled. Suggested potency 30c three times daily for ten days.

**3. ACIDUM NITRICUM** Warts which need this remedy for treatment are long, dark and pointed. They bleed easily and are particularly prominent around the teat orifice. Suggested potency 1m one dose daily for ten days.

**FOOTNOTE** The daily application of an ointment containing Causticum and Thuja will aid the healing process.


# HEAT STRESS

Prolonged exposure to strong sunlight may lead to this condition when the animal becomes restless, exhibiting signs of respiratory distress. The remedies **ACONITUM** 1m and **BELLADONNA** 1m given three times per day in alternation for two days will help alleviate.

# Mastitis

This term loosely covers any condition affecting the mammary gland including bacterial involvement. It can vary from acute inflammations to milder cases showing varying degrees of tissue damage.

The condition is usually brought about by a combination of factors such as faulty management, bacterial infection and injuries. The infective agents are attributable to various strains of Streptococci, Staphylococci, E. coli, Corynebacteria and Pasteurella. Staphylococci are commonly involved where prolonged use of antibiotics has produced resistant strains of Streptococci. The precise role of bacteria as primary causes of mastitis has not been fully determined, but other factors which appear to be of importance are unable to produce the condition in the absence of bacteria. These factors must therefore be considered only to be predisposing. Acute, sub-acute and chronic forms occur.

## CLINICAL SIGNS

General symptoms include changes in milk secretion resulting in abnormalities such as clots and changes in the size and consistency of the udder tissue. There is frequently also a systemic reaction.

**A. ACUTE FORM**   This usually appears as a sequel to kidding and also to a lesser degree at drying off. The onset is usually sudden and the condition can be recognised by swelling of the udder and changes in the milk. The swelling may take several forms ranging from slight oedema to a hot painful enlargement. Hyperacute forms show blood in the milk with a cold udder when systemic changes take place yielding a high temperature and cessation of normal body functions.

**B. CHRONIC FORM**   This also includes what are known as mild cases when feverish symptoms are usually absent. The udder shows fibrous induration in the region of the milk cistern and the milk contains small clots.

*Mastitis caused by Streptococci.* Various species are recognised e.g. S. agalactiae, S. dysgalactiae, and S. pyogenes. The condition is less common in well managed flocks. S. agalactiae is associated with normally mild cases, S. dysgalactiae may yield a more acute syndrome with severe swelling of the udder and changes in milk while systemic involvement may be slight.

*Mastitis caused by Staphylococci.* S. aureus and S. pyogenes are the species most commonly involved. A per-acute form may appear a day or two after kidding which can be fatal, the udder becoming swollen and purple with rapid systemic involvement. The chronic form of this type is characterised by a slowly developing induration of udder tissue with watery secretion leading eventually to atrophy of the secreting tissue of the udder. A form in between the per-acute and chronic forms may yield secretion of a purulent nature containing many thick clots.

## THE ROLE OF HOMOEOPATHY IN MASTITIS CONTROL

When advising an owner with this end in view we stress the importance of tackling the problem on a flock basis rather than seeking out one or two offending animals and treating them individually (see below). In considering prevention we must take account of the various bacteriological influences and if possible employ the appropriate nosode. By first determining which type of mastitis is present in the flock we can easily have a nosode or oral vaccine prepared against the organism concerned. This prior determination is important inasmuch as there is a multiplicity of bacteria capable of being implicated and we cannot always assume we are dealing with one of the commoner types we have mentioned.

For the purpose of flock medication we usually employ the nosode in the 30c potency. Various forms of administration are available depending on individual circumstances e.g. whether the flock is large or small. Large numbers of goats may need to be medicated by giving the nosode in liquid form in the field whereas small numbers or individual animals can be treated orally.

## TREATMENT OF INDIVIDUAL CASES

All outbreaks of mastitis call for the employment of various remedies according to the different symptoms presented, viz the doe's reaction to the condition. Among the commoner remedies used might be the following:

**1. ACONITUM** This remedy should be employed early in acute cases, especially those showing sudden onset and possibly after exposure to cold dry winds. It will allay tension and ease pain. Suggested potency 10m one dose every hour for three doses.

**2. BELLADONNA** This remedy is indicated in the acute form when the udder shows redness and swelling. Pain is obvious on palpation and the skin is hot. Dilated pupils may be seen. Suggested potency 1m one dose every hour for four doses.

**3. APIS MEL.** This is a useful remedy for freshly kidded does showing oedema of the udder and surrounding tissues. Suggested potency 6c one dose every hour for five doses.

**4. BRYONIA** This remedy is indicated where the udder is hard and indurated. In acute cases pain and discomfort will be relieved by pressure on the udder. The animal may be seen lying down. Suggested potency 30c one every two hours for five doses.

**5. ARNICA** Indicated when mastitis develops as a result of injury to the mammary tissue. Blood may be present in the milk. Suggested potency 30c three times daily for three days.

**6. BELLIS PERENNIS** Somewhat similar in its indications to Arnica but more likely to be of benefit if mastitis supervenes after a prolonged or difficult kidding. Suggested potency 30c three times daily for three days.

**7. PHYTOLACCA** This is a very useful remedy both for the acute and chronic forms. Acute cases show clots in the milk while chronic ones show small clots in mid lactation, which is often referred to as sub-clinical. Suggested potency for acute cases one dose three times daily for three days followed by one daily for four days. Sub-clinical cases will possibly require one dose three times daily for seven days.

**8. S.S.C.** This remedy is a combination of Sulphur, Silicea and Carbo Veg. and has been proved in practice to be an excellent remedy for the control of both acute and sub-clinical cases. Clots are usually large and have a yellowish tinge. Suggested potency 30c one three times daily for five days.

**9. HEPAR SULPH.** In low potency this remedy will help promote suppuration in those cases where abscess may have developed. Pain is evident on pressure. Suggested potency 12c one dose every two hours for five doses.

**10. CALCAREA FLUORICA** In those chronic cases showing induration and sterile udder secretion this remedy may prove beneficial. It is a very useful tissue remedy in general. Suggested potency 30c one dose three times per week for four weeks.

**11. SILICEA** Chronic cases showing fistulous involvement and a tendency for infection to break out in different parts of the udder may benefit from this remedy. Suggested potency 200c one dose twice weekly for four weeks.

**12. TUB. BOV.** This nosode has proved useful in those cases showing lumpy induration of the udder giving it a lopsided appearance. The tissues feel doughy. Suggested potency 200c one does per week for four weeks.

# BLOOD IN MILK

Frequently in heavy milkers the milk after kidding may show a pink discolouration or less frequently frank expressions of blood and clots. This can be caused by the pressure in the udder affecting small blood vessels which rupture. Various remedies may be needed to correct the condition chief among them being **ARNICA** 30c or **IPECAC** 6c given three times daily for seven days. If these fail to give satisfactory results remedies such as **FICUS** 6c, **MELILOTUS** 30c, **MILLEFOLIUM** 30c or **CROTALUS** 12c may be needed.

# INJURIES TO TEATS

As in cattle and sheep the teats may be subjected to injuries of various kinds. Sores and cuts may be the source of more serious udder involvement and should be treated by the frequent application of **HYPERCAL** lotion using a dilution of 1/10 in warm water. This is a combination of

**HYPERICUM** and **CALENDULA** and is probably the best healing agent available. See also chapter on wounds and first aid.

# DEFICIENCY OF MILK

This frequently accompanies specific conditions and when these are treated the condition may right itself. Deficiency not associated with any such condition e.g. reduced output after kidding should be helped by one or other of the following remedies:

**1. URTICA URENS** This remedy in high potency e.g. 200c will help stimulate secretion. It should be given twice daily for three days.

**2. AGNUS CASTUS** There may be an accompanying vaginal discharge associated with this remedy. Suggested potency 6c three times daily for seven days.

**3. ASAFOETIDA** This remedy is associated with superficial pain in the udder shown by sensitivity to slight touch. It may be especially useful in the first kidder. Suggested potency 6c one three times daily for five days.

# EXCESS MILK SECRETION

To help dry off the milk the following remedies should be tried:

**1. URTICA URENS** In low potency e.g. 6c this remedy has proved useful giving one dose four times daily for five days.

**2. GALEGA** This is a good remedy also especially in those cases showing digestive weakness and a tendency to anaemia. Suggested potency 6c three times daily for five days.

**3. MEDUSA** This remedy has a strong action on the mammary glands and in 6c potency may help to reduce excess secretion of milk. A dose three times daily for five days should suffice.

# Metabolic Diseases

## 1. LAMINITIS

As in the case of horses and cattle, goats also are subject to this painful condition which by definition is an inflammation of the sensitive laminae within the hoof. It is constitutional in origin.

*CLINICAL SIGNS*
Various forms are recognised ranging from mild to very acute. The classic picture of an animal suffering from laminitis comprises sudden onset, fear, tension and severe pain, together with hot skin, dilated pupils and a full pulse. Together these represent a picture of two separate remedies.

*TREATMENT*
**1. ACONITUM**  This remedy should be given first as soon as possible using a 1m potency one dose every hour for four doses.
**2. BELLADONNA**  The following day this remedy should be given using a potency of 1m daily for five days.
   In the great majority of acute cases the use of these two remedies will bring about resolution and cure.
   Chronic laminitis, is seen in animals which are subject to recurrence, the main remedy to consider being *CALCAREA FLUORICA* 30c. This is an excellent tissue remedy and will alleviate any stress on the laminae and help prevent relapses. A dose three times per week for four weeks should suffice.

## 2. MILK FEVER – HYPOCALCAEMIA

As in cattle this remedy arises post partum when lactation begins. The calcium demands of the kid(s) in utero bring about a depletion of the doe's calcium reserves leading to the onset of the condition in the susceptible animal. It is not particularly common in the goat, and the onset after kidding follows no particular pattern.

## CLINICAL SIGNS
The element calcium has an intricate association with the metabolism of muscle and any disturbance of this leads to a picture of muscle weakness e.g. inability to rise and also to muscle tremors. Normal body functions are interfered with. In mild cases the doe may remain standing but shows unsteadiness and incoordination. Temperature is usually sub-normal.

## TREATMENT
The intravenous use of selected calcium products is usually all that is needed but to prevent relapse and hasten recovery the following remedies will be found useful:

**1. CALCAREA PHOS. and MAGNESIUM PHOSPH.** This combination will help stabilise the calcium and magnesium elements and prevent further loss from the body's reserves. Suggested potency 30c giving a dose three times daily for seven days.

**2. BELLADONNA** If there are signs of disturbance to the central nervous system such as head shaking, excitement or dilated pupils this remedy will help. Suggested potency 1m three times daily for two days.

**3. CONIUM** Recumbent cases showing an inability to rise will be greatly helped by this remedy. Suggested potency 200c three times daily for four days.

# 3. ACETONAEMIA

Sometimes referred to as Ketosis this condition arises from a disturbance of the glycogenic function of the liver, brought about by interference with carbohydrate metabolism. It appears shortly after parturition and is seen particularly in the winter months when does are housed. Acetone bodies called Ketones circulate in the blood and these are responsible for many of the symptoms including the characteristic sweet smell although this is not always apparent.

## CLINICAL SIGNS

There is at first loss of appetite when the animal shows indifference to certain foodstuffs especially concentrates. Nervous symptoms occasionally are seen such as hyper excitability.

## TREATMENT

**1. LYCOPODIUM** This is one of the main remedies in controlling the digestive form of this trouble when inappetance is combined with firm stools having a shiny coating. It produces a tonic effect on the liver helping to regulate the glycogenic function, and restoring normal glucose levels in the blood. Suggested potency 1m one dose daily for ten days.

**2. FLOR DE PIEDRA** This is also a useful remedy acting in much the same way as the previous remedy. It is more suited to the case which tends to relapse. Suggested potency 30c giving a dose three times daily for five days.

**3. NUX VOM.** When acute symptoms have been overcome the use of this remedy will help restore normal digestive function. Suggested potency 1m one dose daily for seven days.

**4, ACONITUM** This remedy should help alleviate the nervous form. It will help calm the doe and reduce any excitement. Suggested potency 1m one dose every hour for four doses.

**5. CICUTA VIROSA** This is a useful remedy for some cases showing nervous complications such as lateral deviation of the neck or pressing the head backwards. Suggested potency 30c one dose three times daily for five days.

# 4. HYPOMAGNESAEMIA

Sometimes referred to as Grass Tetany this condition arises as a result of a sudden fall in the level of magnesium in the blood. There is some doubt about the true cause some authorities considering that the related trace elements Phosphorus and Potassium are implicated as well; an imbalance of these two triggering the fall in magnesium. Fortunately the problem in goats is less severe than the corresponding condition in cattle and sheep.

## CLINICAL SIGNS

Onset is invariably rapid when the animal shows excitability and may stagger, occasionally falling to the ground. Milder cases show muscle tremors over the shoulder and flank. There is a seasonal incidence, spring and autumn being the times when it is most likely to occur.

## TREATMENT

While calcium and magnesium injections are recognised as standard treatment and should always be administered, the following remedies will aid recovery and limit damage to the central nervous system:

**1. CUPRUM ACETICUM**   This is a useful remedy for the milder case which comes on suddenly and is associated with spasm of muscles. If given early it may well prevent the onset of convulsions. Suggested potency 30c three times daily for three days.

**2. GELSEMIUM**   This remedy is helpful in those cases showing muscle tremors and an inability to rise. Frothy mucus is frequently seen around the nostrils and breathing is laboured. Suggested potency 200c one dose every hour for three doses.

**3. MAGNESIUM PHOS.**   This remedy should always be given along with other selected remedies. It will help stabilise the magnesium blood levels. Suggested potency 30c one dose every two hours for four doses.

**4. BELLADONNA** If a more serious case arises (which is uncommon) the use of this remedy will help limit any damage to the central nervous system. Suggested potency 200c giving one dose every hour for four doses.

# 5. ACIDOSIS

This is a condition which is brought on by stasis of the contents of the rumen, consequent on overfeeding especially of concentrates. The fermentation associated with this takes the form of a build up of acid products. Animals which are on a high concentrate diet are less likely to succumb inasmuch as the rumen has adapted to this state of affairs. The goats which are more at risk are those which are already feeding on less productive feed.

## CLINICAL SIGNS

Enlargement of the rumenal area is obvious and palpation reveals the contents to be doughy in character. Erratic movements occurs such as staggering and shaking the head. Pain and distress are obvious. Extreme cases show recumbency when prognosis must be guarded. Looseness of bowels is sometimes present but this does little to relieve the condition.

## TREATMENT

Apart from surgical interference to remove the rumenal contents which is helpful in many instances, the following remedies should be tried:

**1. ACONITUM**   This remedy should be given as soon as the symptoms appear.

**2. NUX VOMICA**   This remedy has a stimulating effect on the digestive organs and should speed the passage of rumenal contents to the other stomachs. Suggested potency 1m one every two hours for four doses.

**3. COLCHICUM**   The fermentation associated with this condition should be helped by this remedy. Suggested potency 30c one dose every hour for four doses.

**4. CARBO VEG.**   In recumbent and serious cases the use of this remedy will help the patient to revive if the condition has not gone too far. Suggested potency 200c one dose every half-hour for four doses.

# 6. PREGNANCY TOXAEMIA

As in sheep this metabolic condition arises in the later stages of pregnancy in susceptible does. It is difficult to treat and the owner should be encouraged to aim at prevention if at all possible, through proper management and feed. Does carrying twins are more at risk because of the extra demands on the dam's system to provide nutrients. Because of the imbalance of the carbohydrate metabolism associated with the condition, breakdown products known as Ketones enter the blood stream and are responsible for many of the symptoms.

## CLINICAL SIGNS

The owner's attention is first drawn to the animal standing apart from the others. Because of the impairment of sight which develops the doe may wander into any object. There is a reluctance to move, while nervous involvement may lead to hyperexcitability.

## TREATMENT

The following remedies may help relieve the condition in those cases which have not gone too far. If the liver has been severely damaged by fatty degeneration treatment may be unsatisfactory.

**1. PHOSPHORUS** This remedy has a beneficial effect on liver function and if the condition is not too far advanced may help resolve it. Suggested potency 200c one dose daily for ten days.

**2. LYCOPODIUM** In mild cases the use of this remedy will help the glycogenic function of the liver and help convert the imbalance brought about by factors leading to the appearance of Ketones in the blood. Suggested potency 1m one daily for ten days.

**3. MAGNESIUM PHOS.** Nervous symptoms such as twitching and muscle tremors should be helped by this remedy. Suggested potency 30c twice daily for ten days.

**PREVENTION** Preventive measures include feeding the doe a liberal amount of good hay together with concentrates in the six weeks of pregnancy.

# 7. OSTEODYSTROPHIA FIBROSA

This condition is associated with two separate elements viz. phosphorus and calcium. It arises when there is an excess of the former over the latter. Young growing kids are at risk when this imbalance is present in the feed.

## CLINICAL SIGNS

The bones, especially of the head become decalcified giving a swollen appearance, spongy to the touch. Other parts of the skeleton can also be affected.

## TREATMENT

The remedy **CALC PHOSPH** should be employed in 30c

potency giving one dose three times per week for six weeks. All young growing kids should be given a preventive dose one per week for three months in an attempt to prevent it arising.

# 8. SWAYBACK.
## Enzootic Ataxia.

This condition is considered to be caused by a deficiency of copper at some stage of the young kid's development.

### CLINICAL SIGNS
The classic picture is one of weak hind-limb movement e.g. inability to raise the hind quarters or weakness generally of that area. Severe cases may show paraplegia.

### TREATMENT
**1. CONIUM** This is a most useful remedy for treatment of mild cases of hind-limb weakness. Suggested potency 30c twice daily for ten days. If this helps it may be necessary to carry on with higher potencies weekly for four weeks e.g. 200c for four weeks, then 1m for four.
**2. LATHYRUS** This also is a useful remedy for mild paralysis affecting forelimbs as well as hind. Suggested potency 1m one daily for fourteen days.
**3. SULFONAL** Animals which keep their feet but present a staggering gait with a tendency to fall sideways may be helped by this remedy. Suggested potency 30c three times daily for ten days.
**PREVENTIVE MEASURES** These include the administration of copper supplements to the doe during pregnancy. From the homoeopathic point of view the use of **CUPRUM METALLICUM** 30c three times per week to the dam for the last six weeks will in some measure help to prevent the condition arising in the kid.

# 9. COBALT DEFICIENCY – PINE

This mineral deficiency is closely associated with the Vitamin B12, which is dependant for its production on an adequate supply of cobalt in the system. The name 'Pine' has come into general use due to the clinical picture of an animal suffering from cobalt deficiency viz. wasting and general unthriftiness.

## CLINICAL SIGNS
Apart from loss of condition, dehydration and dry coat are seen. Anaemia occurs due to the impairment of the B12 metabolism.

## TREATMENT
Either metallic cobalt (**COBALTUM**) or its chloride (**COBALTUM CHLOR.**) should be given using a 30c potency daily for eight weeks. Vitamin B12 supplements should also be given.
**PREVENTION** Cobalt in homoeopathic potency as above should be given as a routine to all goats which graze on land which is cobalt deficient. These areas are to be found in the north-eastern Highlands and in certain islands off the West coast of Scotland, and also in some parts of South West England.


# 10. IODINE DEFICIENCY

The hormone of the thyroid gland depends for its normal production on the element Iodine, lack of which can lead to goitre or swelling of the gland.

## CLINICAL SIGNS
If this hormone is missing or in short supply animals may present with a dry coat, sparse hair and enlarged thyroid gland seen as a swelling on the lower neck area. A tendency to obesity may be seen in long-standing neglected cases.

## TREATMENT
Any procedure which entails the use of iodine compounds will help correct the condition. Homoeopathically this can be achieved by using **IODUM** 30c giving one dose per day for ten days. The remedy **FLOR DE PIEDRA** has an affinity with the thyroid gland and can be used as a follow-up remedy after the iodine metabolism has been stabilised by the administration of **IODUM** 30c. It should be given twice weekly for six weeks.

# 11. RICKETS

This condition arises when there is a deficiency of Vitamin D or when there is a disturbance of the calcium/ phosphorus ratio.

## *CLINICAL SIGNS*
Enlargement of joints occurs following a period of muscular weakness or stiffness, the front legs being more commonly affected. The bones of the rib cage are also affected.

## *TREATMENT*
The following two remedies will cover most ordinary cases encountered:
**1. CALCAREA PHOS.** Young animals should be given a potency of 30c three times per week for six weeks.
**2. PHOSPHORIC ACID** This is also a useful remedy for the growing kid. Suggested potency 30c one dose daily for fourteen days.

# 12. VITAMIN E DEFICIENCY

This is also known as Selenium deficiency as this element is closely associated with Vitamin E metabolism. Under normal circumstances does feeding on a good balanced diet with the proper proportion of minerals and vitamins are unlikely to produce kids showing a deficiency of Selenium or Vitamin E. Does in late pregnancy which are given a subsistence diet lacking in adequate amounts of minerals and other trace elements are more likely to produce susceptible kids.

## *CLINICAL SIGNS*
Both acute and mild manifestations of this deficiency may be met with. The former usually affects the heart muscle and animals may be found dead without showing any symptoms of illness. Vitamin E and Selenium are linked to muscle metabolism and nearly all cases of deficiency show muscle involvement of one kind or another. Mild cases show muscular stiffness and weakness. Animals may become recubent and care should be taken to differenti-

ate this condition from other mineral deficiencies e.g. calcium.

## TREATMENT

The administration of selenium by injection or Vitamin E capsules is normally sufficient to ensure a good response. Homoeopathic treatment to supplement this is based on the remedies **CURARE** 30c, once daily for ten days. **MAGNESIUM PHOSPH.** 30c at the same rate and **CUPRUM METALLICUM** 30c also once daily.

# 13. DEGENERATIVE JOINT DISEASE

This condition may be encountered in bucks which are housed and which are fed on excessive amounts of calcium rich foods. This produces joint lesions such as arthritis and general stiffness when the animal shows disinclination to move around. Treatment should follow the lines as laid down for the control of osteodystrophia which should correct the calcium imbalance. Remedies such as **BRYONIA** 30c, **CALCIUM CARBONATE** 30c and **HECLA LAVA** 200c could all be indicated in treatment depending on overall symptoms.

# Specific Diseases

These are diseases which are identified with bacterial, viral or protozool agents and vary in severity and frequency of occurrence as well as distribution. Not all the ones dealt with here are significant from the point of view of owners in the U.K. but are mentioned as a matter of interest.

## A. DISEASES CAUSED BY BACTERIA
## 1. ENTEROTOXAEMIA

This condition is associated with bacteria of the clostridial family, and causes a serious intestinal disease especially in young kids. Systemic symptoms soon appear after exposure to infection resulting in high temperature, severe diarrhoea and loss of appetite. The condition is not easy to treat but the remedies **PYROGEN** in 1m potency and **ARNSENICUM ALBUM** 1m may give relief in mild cases.

   **PYROGEN** is needed when there is a discrepancy between pulse and temperature e.g. a high pulse alternating with a weak pulse or vice versa.

   **ARSENICUM** may be needed when stools are dark and blood-stained the animals is restless and thirst is evident for small quantities of water.

   The aim in this condition is to achieve prevention and this is normally done by clostridial vaccination. The commercial vaccines available are well proven and give good immunity. Where small numbers of goats are at risk e.g. up to ten animals it is possible to achieve protection homoeopathically by a combined nosode using it in 30c potency and giving one dose twice weekly for four weeks. This should be repeated after two months.

# 2. TETANUS

This disease which is caused by a sporulating anaerobic bacterium called Clostridium tetani is occasionally met with, more especially in kids.

## CLINICAL SIGNS

The owner's attention is first drawn to the young animal walking in an unsteady manner. Examination reveals muscle stiffness and protrusion of the third eyelid occurs. Severe cases involve the central nervous system when convulsions may take place and death supervenes on respiratory failure.

## TREATMENT

This is by no means easy but the following remedies may give some relief and hopefully in mild cases lead to a cure if started early:

**1. ACONITUM**   The fear and anxiety which kids may display calls for the early use of this remedy. Suggested potency 10m one dose every hour for four doses.

**2. CURARE**   This remedy prepared from arrow poison has given good results in cases where muscle stiffness is prominent. Suggested potency 30c giving one dose three times daily for seven days.

**3. STRYCHNINUM**   The arching of the back together with extension of limbs and head provides a picture which is relevant to this remedy. High potencies should be considered e.g. 200c twice daily for three days, followed by 1m daily for ten days.

**4. HYPERICUM**   This remedy should, if disease is suspected provide help in limiting the spread of the toxin. Suggested potency 1m three times daily for seven days.

**5. LEDUM**   Along with the previous remedy, Ledum will help materially in the early stages. It is the prime remedy to consider in treatment of punctured wounds although it must be stressed that not all cases of tetanus show obvious penetration of skin. Many cases are what are known as idiopathic where no signs of external wounds can be found. Suggested potency 6c giving one dose three times daily for seven days along with the previous remedy.

**6. TETANUS NOSODE**   The combination of nosode

and selected remedy is always useful, giving a daily dose of 30c for seven days.

# 3.  COLI-BACILLOSIS:
## White or Dietary Scour

This condition is associated with a disturbance of the E. Coli function in the intestine. This bacterium plays an essential role in maintaining a healthy bowel flora and causes disease only when the animal is put under some form of stress e.g. exposure to prolonged wet or cold or deprivation of colostrum after birth.

### *CLINICAL SIGNS*
Kids may appear normal at birth but can quickly show signs of shock viz. cold muzzle, sub-normal temperature, cold extremities and rapid weak pulse. This is soon followed by whitish or yellow pasty faeces soon becoming liquid and often preceded by abdominal bloating. The motions have a characteristic sickly odour. Sudden prostration can occur and is a serious development. Fever is usually absent. A frequent sequel is pneumonia due to septicaemic complications.

Kids which are deprived of colostrum are particularly at risk as are those which are subjected to severe weather conditions.

### *TREATMENT*
**1.  ACONITUM**   The early use of this remedy will help allay shock and anxiety, especially in those cases which show a sudden onset. Suggested potency 1m one dose every hour for four doses.
**2.  VERATRUM ALB.**   With this remedy there is a general appearance of collapse with signs of abdominal pain preceding the onset of scour. Stools are watery and forcibly expelled, while body sweating may occur. The kid is cold and visible mucous membranes have a bluish tinge. Suggested potency 30c one dose every two hours for four doses.
**3.  PULSATILLA**   When this remedy is indicated it will be found that the character of the stool changes frequently e.g. at one stage it may contain a significant amount of mucus while at others it may be watery. Changeability of symptoms and thirstlessness is a keynote

of this remedy. Suggested potency 30c one three times daily for five days.

**4. CARBO VEG.** Stools are preceded by signs of abdominal colic and flatulence. It is an excellent remedy for helping to revive apparently moribund patients. Such kids should be given access to a plentiful supply of fresh air. Suggested potency 200c one dose every hour for four doses.

**5. PYROGEN** This is one of the most valuable remedies to employ when septicaemic complications arise characterised by discrepancies between pulse and temperature. There is usually a putrid odour to the stool. Suggested potency 1m one dose every two hours for four doses.

**6. DULCAMARA** This is a good remedy if the onset of disease is associated with exposure to damp or excessive wetting. Kids born in the autumn are more likely to need this remedy than those born in the spring. Suggested potency 200c one twice daily for five days.

**7. CAMPHORA** This is another remedy which is associated with collapsed states. There is extreme coldness of body and mouth while motions may be passed involuntarily. Suggested potency 6c one dose every hour for six doses.

**8. CHINA** This remedy is of great value in helping to restore strength after loss of body fluid. It will also help control diarrhoea. Suggested potency 6c one dose every two hours for four doses.

**9. E. COLI NOSODE** It has been found in practice that the use of this nosode provides rapid relief if not too long delayed. Suggested potency 30c one three times daily for two days.

**PREVENTION** If the E. coli nosode is administered at birth and again at 24, 48 and 72 hours it will greatly reduce the chance of infection arising.

# 4. NAVEL ILL OR JOINT ILL

Unhygienic conditions can lead to the development of this condition. Not all forms of navel ill lead to joint ill and the latter can exist independently of apparent umbilical connection.

## CLINICAL SIGNS

The umbilicus becomes swollen and spongy and in white breeds shows red due to inflammation. Systemic involvement leads to inappetance and, if joints become affected, to swelling and pain in various joints. E. coli organisms and various strains of Streptococci are usually incriminated. The carpal (knee) joint is mostly affected.

## TREATMENT

**1. ACONITUM**   This should be given early as in other febrile conditions. Suggested potency 1m one dose every hour for four doses.

**2. BRYONIA**   Joints appear swollen and hot. Movement aggravates any pain present while pressure on the joint relieves pain. Suggested potency 6c one dose three times daily for five days.

**3. RUTA**   This remedy will relieve any distress associated with inflammation of periosteum and surrounding areas of the joints. Suggested potency 1m one dose daily for seven days.

**4. LEDUM**   This remedy should help relieve symptoms associated with shoulder and fetlock areas. Suggested potency 30c three times daily for five days.

**5. BENZOIC ACID**   The hock and tendons down to the Achilles area are involved when this remedy is indicated. Heat and swelling appear on these areas. Suggested potency 6c one dose three times daily for five days.

**6. STREPTOCOCCUS NOSODE**   This remedy has given good results in practice and can be used along with other remedies. Suggested potency 30c three times daily for three days.

# 5. FOOT ROT

This condition is caused by an organism called Fusiformis nodosus which contaminates soil in damp or marshy areas. It is extremely common in sheep under prevailing conditions and can affect goats to a lesser degree.

## CLINICAL SIGNS

Slight lameness is an early sign and depending on conditions and virulence varying degrees of involvement are seen. Severe cases manifest themselves by extreme lameness a common sight being the animal grazing by resting on its knees, thereby avoiding contact with the ground by the affected foot. The horn of the hoof becomes soft and crumbly and gives off an unpleasant odour. Constitutional involvement may lead to loss of condition and in does a fall in milk yield.

## TREATMENT
The following remedies have all proved useful:
**1. KREOSOTUM**   This is one of the main remedies. It has a profound action on diseased horn and surrounding tissues. Suggested potency 200c one dose twice weekly for four to six weeks.
**2. HEPAR SULPH.**   The pain associated with the condition should be relieved by this remedy as this is one of the keynotes for its use in infected states. Suggested potency 1m daily for seven days.
**3. SILICEA**   Once the acute state has been relieved this remedy should follow as it will quickly build up hard healthy horn which will more easily resist subsequent infection. Suggested potency 200c one dose twice weekly for six weeks.
**4. FOOT ROT NOSODE**   As a complementary measure the nosode should be employed using a 30c potency daily for seven days.
**PREVENTION**   A 30c potency of the nosode should be given at the beginning of autumn and again in the spring administering it twice weekly for six weeks.


# 6.  SEEDY TOE

This bacterial condition is occasionally met with caused by invasion of pus producing bacteria leading to purulent discharges around the coronet.

## CLINICAL SIGNS
Lameness is obvious and the infective process is seen as purulent material oozing from the coronary band at the junction of hoof and skin.

## TREATMENT
The following remedies have all proved useful in practice:

**1. HEPAR SULPH.**  In the early acute (painful) stage this remedy will be of great benefit. A high potency e.g. 200c should be considered giving a dose daily for seven days.

**2. MYRISTICA**  This is another very useful remedy in the less acute case. It has a strong action on septic conditions associated with the feet. Suggested potency 30c giving a dose twice daily for ten days.

**3. SILICEA**  This remedy should be considered in chronic cases. Apart from its value in treating septic conditions it will harden the horn and promote healthy growth. Suggested potency 200c one dose twice weekly for six weeks.

**4. CALCAREA FLUORICA**  Any spongy tissue remaining above the coronary band after treatment will heal under the influence of this remedy. Suggested potency 30c twice weekly for six weeks.

**5. HYPERCAL LOTION**  This lotion diluted 1/10 in warm water will have a healing effect locally applied. The parts should be bathed two or three times daily if possible.


# 7. LEPTOSPIROSIS

This disease is relatively uncommon as an acute condition but reports from abroad suggest that sub-clinical disease is not uncommon. This frequently takes the form of anorexic weakness and impairment of kidney function. Haemoglobinuria is occasionally seen but abortions are uncommon.

Treatment is frequently unsatisfactory as the disease has a rapidly fatal outcome. The most useful approach would be an attempt to control the disease by the use of the appropriate nosode. This could easily be done by employing the particular strain of Leptospira involved, taking blood from an infected animal as the source. This could then be given on a flock basis twice weekly for eight weeks using a 30c potency.


# 8. JOHNE'S DISEASE

This disease is associated with gradual loss of weight following infection of the intestinal mucosa by a bacillus known as Mycobacterium Johnei. It is prevalent world wide. There is a long incubation period, young goats which become infected showing symptoms anything up to eighteen months later.

## CLINICAL SIGNS
Emaciation develops gradually. Bowel movements tend to be soft, but watery diarrhoea as seen in cattle is relatively uncommon. Does in milk gradually cease production.

## TREATMENT
This is likely to be unsatisfactory in the great majority of cases but one or two animals have shown a response to selected remedies, although even in these cases relapses are common.

**1. ACID NIT.** This remedy has helped some cases of colitis and may control the condition by restoring tone to the intestinal mucosa. Suggested potency 200c one dose three times per week for four weeks.

**2. ALOE** There may be signs of pain or rectal irritation if this remedy is indicated. Stools are blood-stained and contain mucus. Suggested potency 30c daily for fourteen days.

**3. GAERTNER** The use of this bowel nosode is indicated in the younger animal. It has a stimulating effect on the bowel mucosa. Suggested potency 30c one dose daily for seven days.

**4. JOHNE'S DISEASE NOSODE** This should aid the action of other remedies and can be given daily for seven days in a 30c potency.

**PREVENTION** The nosode should be given on a flock basis where infection has occurred. One dose of 30c potency should be given to each animal twice weekly for six weeks. This may help build up a measure of protection.


# 9. ENZOOTIC PNEUMONIA (PASTEURELLOSIS)

This condition usually presents as a broncho-pneumonia. There is some doubt as to whether this disease is a primary phenomenon, some authorities believing that it is secondary to an underlying viral or mycoplasma infection. As in sheep, predisposing factors include stress such as over-crowding and lack of proper ventilation among housed animals.

## CLINICAL SIGNS
Early fever and distressed breathing are followed by inappetance and frequent coughing which is usually dry and rasping. Very acute cases can die quickly without warning. Fall of milk yield occurs in lactating does. Purulent discharges may develop accompanied by grunting.

## TREATMENT
The following remedies should be considered:

**1. FERRUM PHOS.**   This is a most useful remedy for feverish conditions of the respiratory tract. Suggested potency 30c one dose every hour for four doses.

**2. PHOSPHORUS**  This is indicated when there is rapid involvement of lung tissue shown by very distressed and laboured breathing. A rust coloured sputum is sometimes coughed up. Suggested potency 200c three times daily for two days.

**3. BRYONIA**   This remedy is indicated when the animal is disinclined to move. If recumbent the patient lies on the affected side. Suggested potency 30c three times daily for seven days.

**4. BERYLLIUM**  This metallic remedy has proved useful in many illnesses where coughing is a prominent symptom. It is indicated especially when the underlying condition is more severe than clinical findings would suggest. Suggested potency 30c three times daily for four days.

**5. TUB. AVIARE**  When the upper portions of the lungs are more involved than the lower. Young animals respond especially well. Suggested potency 200c once daily for ten days.

**6. DROSERA**   The type of cough suggesting this remedy is spasmodic in nature. It has given especially good results in the younger animal. Suggested potency 9c three times daily for seven days.

**7. ANTIMONIUM ARSENICOSUM**  This remedy should be considered when there is severe dyspnoea. The upper left chest area is affected more than the other areas. The patient prefers to remain standing. Suggested potency 30c three times daily for seven days.

**8. AMMONIUM CAUSTICUM** Severely-laboured breathing is again common with this remedy. Signs of pain or discomfort are seen on breathing, the animal becoming restless, frequently changing position. Suggested potency 30c three times daily for seven days.

# 10. CASEOUS LYMPHADENITIS

This is a chronic condition which is capable of spreading from one goat to another. It is characterised by multiple abscesses which appear in the lymph glands. All age groups can be affected but it is probably more likely to be encountered in the older age group. The causative organism is CORYNEBACTERIUM OVIS.

*CLINICAL SIGNS*
Swellings appear in the regional lymph nodes prediliction sites being the mandibular and parotid glands. Other ones which may become affected are the supramammary and popliteal. Most of the cervical lymph nodes can also be affected in severe outbreaks. Rapid breathing and coughing are signs that deeper lymph nodes are affected. The incubation period is relatively long, up to four months in some cases. Abscesses which develop are referred to as cold or painess and as they mature the skin covering them becomes hairless. Maturation of the abscess yields a pus which is yellowish and sometimes greenish.

*TREATMENT*
There are many useful remedies to consider in controlling the spread of this infection and limiting it within the affected animal. These include:
**1. SILICEA** This is probably the most important remedy being well proven in the treatment of chronic cold abscesses. Suggested potency 200c one three times per week for four weeks.
**2. CALCAREA FLUORICA** The hardness and swelling of the lymph nodes which develop during abscess formation will be aided by this remedy. Suggested potency 30c one daily for ten days.
**3. GUNPOWDER** This remedy has proved useful in the treatment of multiple abscesses and is beneficial in the

early stages of abscess formation. Suggested potency 6c three times daily for five days.

**4. TARENTULA CUBENSIS** Excessive hardness surrounding the abscess with a tendency to necrosis of skin calls for this remedy. Suggested potency 30c three times daily for five days.

**5. PHOSPHORUS** If the supramammary lymph nodes are more prominently affected than others this remedy may help. Suggested potency 200c one three times per week for four weeks.

**6. MERC. SOL.** If the pus is greenish this is a keynote of this remedy. It should benefit the submaxillary and parotid glands in particular. Suggested potency 30c one daily for seven days.

**7. C. OVIS NOSODE** This can be prepared from the pus from any gland and after potentising given daily for seven days in a 30c potency. It can be combined with any selected remedy.

**CONTROL** The nosode should be considered as a prophylactic measure in all flocks which are at risk. A twice monthly dose of 30c potency should be given for four months.

# 11. SALMONELLOSIS

This condition is seen more frequently abroad but it has been known to occur in the U.K. Sub-clinical disease can occur when no overt symptoms are presented, but the animal can shed the organism in the faeces. Conditions which produce E. coli infection such as stress and exposure to inclement weather can also precipitate clinical symptoms in Salmonella infections.

## CLINICAL SIGNS
The disease affects mainly young kids which portray severe diarrhoea and fever. Systemic involvement takes the form of a septicaemia. The diarrhoea is frequently blood-stained and because of haemorrhages which take place in the upper intestines, it may appear dark.

## TREATMENT
Septicaemic cases often die before treatment can be started but in milder forms the following remedies are worth trying:

**1. ACONITUM**   Should be given as soon as symptoms appear. Suggested potency 1m one dose every hour for four doses.

**2. ARSENICUM ALB.**   This remedy should help control the dark foul-smelling diarrhoea which occurs. Suggested potency 1m giving one dose every three hours for four doses and repeating once daily for five days.

**3. VERATRUM ALB.**   When collapse is threatened and faeces are forcibly evacuated. Suggested potency 30c one every two hours for four doses.

**4. PYROGEN**   This remedy is particuarly indicated especially when there is a discrepancy between pulse and temperature. Suggested potency 1m one dose every three hours for four doses.

**5. SALMONELLA NOSODE**   This nosode has been prepared against the two main types of Salmonella associated with disease. It can be combined with selected remedies giving a dose of 30c potency daily for seven days.

**PREVENTION**   Kids should be given a daily dose of 30c potency daily for five days and repeated once per week for four weeks.

# B. DISEASES CAUSED BY VIRUSES

Viruses are different from bacteria in that they can penetrate the cells of the body where they replicate and in many instances cause serious disease. Virus diseases as a whole are becoming increasingly important both in the U.K. and elsewhere. We can now examine the main ones which affect the goat population.

# 1. LOUPING ILL

This disease is a meningo-encephalitis affecting the central nervous system and is caused by a vector of the tick family known as Ixodes ricinus. It occurs on upland and hill pastures in spring and autumn when goats and sheep are most at risk from tick activity. The virus is transmitted when the tick bites the animal. Fortunately the disease in goats is much less common than in sheep but it has been known to occur occasionally and would probably be more widespread if goats grazed on infested pastures in the numbers that sheep do.

## CLINICAL SIGNS
Once the disease is established the animal develops a jumpy or hopping gait (hence the name Louping Ill). This is due to erratic stimulation of the nerves of the spinal cord. Severe cases become recumbent when paralysis sets in.

## TREATMENT
Early cases may show a reasonably good response to the following:

**1. AGARICUS** This remedy produces a picture of incoordination sometimes referred to as a "drunken" state. There is a tendency to fall backwards, along with twitching of head muscles. Excitability is seen brought on by an increased response to external stimuli. Suggested potency 30c one three times daily for seven days.

**2. CICUTA VIROSA** Laterial deviation of the head to the right may indicate this remedy with a tendency for the head to be pressed backwards. Muscular spasms occur. Suggested potency 200c one daily for five days.

**3. CONIUM** In mild cases showing weakness of the hind limbs this remedy should help. The paralysis presents as an ascending weakness of nerves from hind limbs upward. The animal rises with difficulty and stumbles frequently. Suggested potency 30c twice daily for fourteen days. Ascending potencies up to 10m may be needed depending on response.

**4. STRAMONIUM** Lateral deviation of the head is again seen with this remedy but to the left with a tendency to fall to that side. Suggested potency 200c one daily for seven days.

**5. LOUPING ILL NOSODE** A useful nosode has been prepared against this disease prepared from infected spinal cord and thereafter potentised. It can be used along with other remedies on a daily basis for seven days.

# 2. CAPRINE ARTHRITIS ENCEPHALITIS

Known simply as CAE this virus disease has been known for only a relatively short time. The virus which causes it is a member of the retrovirus group (associated with diseases such as Feline Leukaemia and Maedi Visna). Young kids are at risk from older infected animals. The young animals may show paralysis while in adults the disease is characterised by arthritis. It is unusual for goats once infected to clear themselves of infection, a carrier state being normal.

## CLINICAL SIGNS

Young kids affected by the encephalitic form show varying symptoms depending on the virulence of the infection e.g. mild cases may present little more than staggering or an uncertain gait, whereas more severe cases rapidly progress to paralysis. Hind-limb weakness is often an early sign but soon all legs become involved within a few weeks.

In the adult animal early arthritis develops and becomes progressively worse. A harsh dry coat develops in the early stages when infected kids grow to maturity. The carpal (or knee) joints are the ones most at risk. Under-lying tissues such as tendon sheaths and ligaments also become involved. Affected joints remain free of secondary infection.

## TREATMENT

This is likely to be of limited value but certain remedies may help in the early stages if given in time.

**1. AGARICUS**  This remedy gives a picture of incoordinated gait and may give some relief in the early paralytic phase. Suggested potency 1m three times daily for five days.

**2. CONIUM**  Early hind-leg weakness will be helped by this remedy possessing as it does a symptom-picture of posterior paralysis extending upwards to other areas. Suggested potency 30c one daily for ten days, followed by 200c three times weekly for four weeks.

**3. STRAMONIUM**  Staggering and falling towards the left side indicates a need for this remedy. Suggested potency 200c three times weekly for four weeks.

**4. CICUTA VIROSA**  Recumbent cases showing a tendency to bend the head backwards or present the neck in a twisted S shaped bend may need this remedy. Suggested potency 30c daily for fourteen days.

**5. RHUS TOX**  If the arthritis state has not progressed

too far this remedy may give some relief. It should be given in 6c potency one dose three times per day for twenty-one days, followed by a potency of 1m three times per week for four weeks.

Other remedies which could also be tried in the early arthritic form are **ACID SALICYLIC** 200c and **GREEN MUSSEL** 200c giving one dose three times per week for four weeks.

**PREVENTION**   A nosode against CAE has been developed and although little or no work has been done to prove its efficacy it is logical to assume that a degree of protection would follow its use, as is the case with other diseases. As the disease is likely to become more prevalent this approach is worth trying. (See Chapter on Vaccination procedure.)

# 3. MAEDI VISNA

This condition is a chronic pneumonia caused by a specific virus. Goats like sheep can be infected at an early age and may now show symptoms for any period up to two years.

## CLINICAL SIGNS
The first sign that something may be wrong is loss of condition accompanied by difficult breathing. Rapid consolidation of lung tissue takes place giving the clinical picture of a severe pneumonia.

## TREATMENT
This is likely to be unrewarding but the following remedies could be tried in mild cases:

**1. FERRUM PHOS.**   This is a most useful remedy for the early treatment of respiratory conditions. Suggested potency 30c three times daily for two days.

**2. PHOSPHORUS** This is a useful remedy in pneumonic cases where consolidation of lung tissue has taken place. Suggested potency 200c twice daily for seven days.

**3. ANTIMONIUM TART.**   This remedy is indicated when there is an excess of mucus present. A moist cough accompanies this. Suggested potency 30c three times daily for seven days.

**4. LYCOPODIUM** In excessively lean animals or

those showing rapid wasting this remedy may help. There may be a late-afternoon aggravation of symptoms and independent movement of the nostrils. Suggested potency 1m twice daily for seven days.

# 4. BLUE TONGUE

This viral disease is transmitted by insects, sheep as well as goats being susceptible. It is not known at present in the U.K. but mention of it is made here to provide goat keepers with a picture which they could recognise.

### *CLINICAL SIGNS*
These include swelling of the lips and a dark discolouration of the mucous membranes of the mouth, the swelling and discolouration extending to the entire head.

It would be possible to have a nosode made against this disease when we would expect a degree of protection to be achieved.

### *TREATMENT*
Would not be allowed under present Ministry regulations in the U.K.

# 5. ORF-CONTAGIOUS PUSTULAR DERMATITIS

This viral disease which also affects sheep is highly contagious and the cause of much unthriftiness in early summer when it is chiefly encountered, although a severe form is occasionally met with in winter during mild wet weather.

Most age groups among the goat population are affected.

### *CLINICAL SIGNS*
Raw bleeding areas appear around the muzzle, these quickly coalescing into large scabby lesions. When these dry the scabs tend to fall off and healing follows. Loss of condition accompanies the process due to the animal's reluctance or inability to feed because of pain around the mouth. Constitutional involvement in milking does lead to reduced milk output.

## TREATMENT

There are useful remedies available and these include the following:

**1. ACID NIT.** This is a prime remedy to consider in any eczematous condition appearing at the junction of skin and any mucous membrane. It will quickly resolve the condition and limit spread. Suggested potency 200c once daily for seven days.

**2. RHUS TOX.** The so-called malignant form of orf which occasionally arises on the udder and surrounding skin in older does should be helped by this remedy. Suggested potency 1m daily for fourteen days.

**3. ORF NOSODE** This is an excellent remedial agent which can be used along with other remedies. It complements their action. Suggested potency 30c one dose daily for five days.

**4. CALENDULA/HYPERICUM LOTION** This lotion, available commercially as **HYPERCAL** will prove a very useful accessory to internal treatment. A dilution of 1/10 should be employed and the lesions bathed a few times daily. Care should be taken to avoid contact with lesions as this condition has been known to be transmissible to susceptible individuals.

**PREVENTION** Orf nosode should be given to all young kids at an early age. A suitable regime would be one dose three times daily for two days followed by one per week for four weeks.

# Miscellaneous
# Specific Conditions

## 1. LISTERIOSIS

Sometimes referred to as Circling Disease this condition is related to the central nervous system and takes various forms ranging from inflammation of the brain to acute septicaemia and abortion. If the encephalitic form attacks a flock it is seldom that the abortion form will be seen in the same group of goats. Shedding of infected material can occur from all body secretions, milk being no exception.

### CLINICAL SIGNS
Encephalitis or circling manifests itself by the patient turning round constantly and may show as head pain by the animal pressing the head against any convenient object. At this stage the head is turned to one side. In the abortion form expulsion of the foetus is confined to the later stages of pregnancy.

### TREATMENT
The following remedies may prove useful in cases which are not too far advanced:
**1. STRAMONIUM** If the circling takes the form of movement from right to left this remedy is indicated. Suggested potency 200c three times per week for four weeks.
**2. CICUTA VIROSA** The reverse state of affairs including lateral deviation of the head to the right or bent backwards calls for this remedy. Suggested potency 30c one daily for ten days.
**3. SULFONAL** Signs of pain or distress are seen if the patient is made to raise the head or have it moved in any way. There is a blood-shot appearance to the eyes. If made to rise the patient exhibits vertigo-like movement such as staggering or incoordination. Suggested potency 30c three times daily for five days.

**4. LISTERIA NOSODE**   This could be made from any affected secretion and used in 30c potency. It should aid the action of selected remedies and can also be used as a prophylactic measure.


# 2. COCCIDIOSIS

This is an important protozoal disease affecting many housed goats, although it can occur under other conditions also. It is caused by various species of the Eimeria family which parasitise the intestinal canal producing what are known as oocysts which pass out in the droppings and after undergoing a definite life cycle are then ready to affect other goats on ingestion of infected material.

## CLINICAL SIGNS
Various forms of virulence are recognised ranging from mild to hyperacute. Mild forms show little more than loose stools, blood being absent. The more acute form presents as a blood-stained or frankly bloody diarrhoea accompanied by severe straining. Dehydration is the normal state of affairs with this. The hyperacute form may yield little or no symptoms, the animal dying within a few hours after ingestion of material containing oocysts.

## TREATMENT
There are reasonaby effective conventional drugs available for the treatment of this condition but if homoeopathic remedies are needed the following will all prove effective in their individual ways, either by themselves or as complementary agents to other measures:
**1. ACONITUM**   If seen in the early stages this remedy may help limit the disease process. Suggested potency 1m one dose every hour for four doses.
**2. ARSENICUM ALBUM**   This remedy should prove effective in the milder case showing diarrhoea and loss of condition with a dry coat and unthrifty appearance. Suggested potency 1m one dose three times daily for four days.
**3. IPECACUANHA**   This is an important remedy for this particular condition. Not only is it a good anti-haemorrhagic remedy in its own right but it appears to have a specific action on the intestine in the presence of

protozoa. Suggested potency 30c one dose three times daily for five days.

**4. MERCURIUS CORR.** This remedy is valuable when there is severe straining accompanying dysenteric slimy stools. Suggested potency 200c twice daily for five days.

**5. CINCHONA (CHINA)** This remedy will help restore strength after loss of body fluid following diarrhoea. Suggested potency 6c three times per day for three days.

**6. VERATRUM ALB.** This remedy should help milder cases showing persistent diarrhoea of an explosive type with threatened collapse. Suggested potency 30c three times daily for five days.

**7. SYCOTIC CO.** This bowel nosode can be given once daily for seven days. It should aid the action of any selected remedy. Potency 30c.

# 3. SCRAPIE

This disease of the nervous system is much less common in goats than in sheep but occasionally it is encountered. Little is known regarding the actual cause but a virus-like agent is thought to be responsible.

## *CLINICAL SIGNS*
An affected animal will first present hyperexcitable behaviour, responding to stimuli by exaggerated movements such as raising the feet and rubbing against any convenient object. Muscle tremors occur around the head and neck. The excessive itching and rubbing eventually leads to hair loss and emaciation. Abnormal mouth movements are sometimes noticed leading to an inability to masticate food properly. As the condition progresses the patient becomes recumbent and death follows.

Treatment is inadvisable but a nosode has been developed against this disease, and although little or no tests have been carried out it could be worth trying as a preventive measure in flocks which have experienced the disease.

# 4. ABORTION AS AN ACCOMPANI-MENT TO SPECIFIC DISEASE

## CHLAMYDIOSIS

This condition also known as ENZOOTIC ABORTION is caused by an infective agent named Chlamydia psittaci. It affects pregnant does giving rise to abortion, the foetus being expelled in late pregnancy. In-kid does are at risk when infected pregnant does are introduced into the flock. Discharges at the time of abortion are heavily contaminated as is the placenta. Does experiencing a mild infection may carry their kids to full term. These young kids then carry the infection themselves and will abort in their first pregnancy. Stillbirths and weak kids are variations on actual miscarriage.

### CLINICAL SIGNS
These are not noticeable until abortion becomes imminent. Post-partum a blood-stained discharge occurs. Accompanying symptoms associated with pneumonia and arthritis may be present: also corneal opacities.

### TREATMENT
This is confined to helping the doe to recover quickly after the expulsion of the foetus. The remedy **SABINA** in 6c potency given three times daily for five days will help clear the vaginal discharge when a significant amount of blood is present. Discharge containing less blood could be helped by **CAULOPHYLLUM** 30c and **SECALE** 30c, again given three times daily for five days. **SEPIA** 200c one daily for three days will aid the general health of the doe and enable the genital tract to recover.
**PREVENTION**   Enzootic abortion nosode is available and should be given to all does whether or not infection is present in the flock. A potency of 30c should be used. (See chapter on vaccination procedure.)

# 5. MYCOPLASMA INFECTION

Various species of the mycoplasma family are responsible for disease in animals causing differing pathological conditions. The ones which should concern us in goats are contagious agalactia, contagious pleuro-pneumonia, multiple arthritis and keratitis.

**1. CONTAGIOUS AGALACTIA.** The clinical signs associated with this complaint vary from acute septicaemia to involvement of udder tissue resulting in mastitis and replacement of milk producing areas with fibrous tissue. Eye lesions are also common ranging from conjunctivitis of varying severity to inflammation of the cornea and iris. Joint lesions also develop.

**2. CONTAGIOUS PLEURO-PNEUMONIA.** This condition has been reported from various parts of Europe. Infection occurs from inhaling respiratory droplets. Pleurisy first develops when rapid breathing occurs with disinclination to move. Untreated cases quickly progress to an acute pneumonia when rust-coloured or blood-stained mucus is coughed up.

**3. MULTIPLE ARTHRITIS INFECTION** This is more common than the preceding forms and follows a septicaemic state. Rapid involvement of joints may result in a high mortality among young goats.

**4. KERATITIS** The clinical picture of this form of mycoplasma infection is not unlike that associated with Kerato-conjunctivitis of sheep and cattle (New Forest Disease). Early symptoms include reddening of the conjunction and cornea which soon becomes opaque. Lachrymation also develops.

*TREATMENTS*

In the agalactia form when the udder becomes affected the remedies listed under the chapter on mastitis should be considered. Pleuritic forms should be helped initially with **BRYONIA** 6c giving a dose three times daily for five days. This should be followed by **FERRUM PHOS** 30c three times daily for three days which will be helpful in delaying the onset of pneumonia. If the latter state develops the remedies **PHOSPHORUS** 200c and **LYCOPODIUM** 1m should be considered three times per week for three weeks. The remedy **ANTIMONIUM ARSENICOSUM** 30c has also been used successfully. Eye conditions will respond satisfactorily to remedies such as **SILICEA** 200c, **CANNABIS SATIVA** 30c, **CALCAREA FLUORICA** 30c, **RUTA** 1m and **LEDUM** 200c depending on overall symptoms presented.

**CONTROL** Depending on which strain of mycoplasma is involved it should be possible to have a nosode prepared and used as a preventive measure as in other specific diseases.

# 6. TOXOPLASMOSIS

This disease while being relatively uncommon in the goat deserves mention because of the potential public health hazard. Goats can become infected by contact with cat faeces or cat placenta, the organism concerned T. Gondii being excreted via the bowel and in the afterbirths. Infected animals present symptoms suggestive of central nervous system disturbance and care must be taken to have such symptoms investigated as they can be indicative of other less serious complaints. Toxoplasma nosode is available as a prophylactic measure and used as in other conditions.

# 7. Q FEVER

This is a zoonotic disease caused by a Rickettsial organism called Coxilla burnetti. Its chief implication for goat keepers lies in its ability to cause abortions and its danger to human beings.

### CLINICAL SIGNS
Although the condition is rare in goats, fever, pneumonia and purulent opthalmia have been known to occur in addition to abortions. The organism can be shed in milk animals which are in contact with pneumonic cases and those which have aborted are themselves at risk of infection.

### TREATMENT
Remedies such as **PHOSPHORUS** 200c, **PYROGEN** 1m, **MERC SOL** and **ARGENTUM NITRICUM** could be tried depending on individual symptoms presented.

# 8. CONTAGIOUS OPTHALMIA: New Forest Disease

This is another Rickettsial disease seen mainly in the

summer months affecting goats kept in unhygienic conditions, but also outside in fields and wooded surroundings. The disease can be spread by flies.

## CLINICAL SIGNS

The condition may attack one or both eyes: after an incubation period of a week the eyes start to water and the conjunctiva become red and inflamed. A white spot develops on the cornea leading eventually to an opaque covering and ulceration. Secondary infection by pyogenic bacteria is common in neglected cases and leads to the development of opthalmia with resulting purulent discharges.

## TREATMENT

It is essential that treatment be started as soon as possible in order to avoid complications.

**1. ACONITUM**   This remedy should be given early. The animal at this stage may be listless with a slightly inflamed eye. Suggested potency 1m one every hour for four doses.

**2. KALI IOD.**   This is also a useful remedy in the early stages when the eye is reddened and lachrymation starts. Suggested potency 200c one dose twice daily for three days.

**3. SILICEA**   This is the remedy of choice once corneal opacity has developed. It will hasten the absorption of scar tissue. Suggested potency 200c one dose three times per week for three weeks.

**4. ACID NITRIC**   If corneal ulceration has developed this remedy may help. Suggested potency 200c one daily for ten days.

**5. ARGENTUM NITRICUM** If opthalmia is threatening with purulent discharges beginning use should be made of this remedy. Suggested potency 30c three times daily for four days.

**6. AN EYE LOTION** containing a combination of **HYPERICUM, CALENDULA** and **CINERARIA** tinctures diluted 1/10 will help externally. The eyes should be bathed with this twice daily.

**PREVENTION**   A good nosode is available as a preventive measure. Goats should be given a dose of 30c potency three times per week for four weeks before the hotter summer months begin e.g. around the beginning of May.

# 9. PARASITIC BRONCHITIS:
## Lungworm Disease

Various species of worm can affect the lungs of goats, some causing overt disease symptoms and others existing in the animal and causing sub-clinical disease.

## CLINICAL SIGNS
Symptoms appear in early summer and again in autumn. Coughing its the first noticeable sign and is usually present in a group of goats in largish flocks. The cough is husky and the animal extends the neck in a characteristic manner with protrusion of the tongue. There is nearly always an abundance of frothy saliva around the mouth. Signs of more severe respiratory distress are soon evident such as laboured breathing especially on exertion. Neglected cases lead on to pulmonary emphysema.

## TREATMENT
Modern anthelmintics are profitaby employed in treatment but there are many useful homoeopathic remedies which can also be given on a constitutional basis which will hasten resolution of the condition. These include:

**1. ANTIMONIUM TART.**  This is indicated when there is an abundance of frothy mucus producing a moist cough. Mucus may be heard rattling in the chest and the cough is worse at night. Suggested potency 30c three times daily for five days.

**2. AMMONIUM CARB.**  This is a useful remedy when pneumonic symptoms are worse in the right lung and the disease is associated with damp weather. Suggested potency 30c one dose three times daily for five days.

**3. ANTIMONIUM ARSENICOSUM**  This remedy is more useful when the left lung is involved and when emphysema has set in. Coughing is worse when the animal is recumbent. Suggested potency 30c three times daily for five days.

**4. ARSENICUM IODATUM**  This is a good remedy to employ in neglected cases when symptoms are aggravated by cold and relieved by warmth. The animal prefers to remain standing finding breathing easier in this position. Suggested potency 6c one dose three times daily for ten days.

**PREVENTION**  A reliable nosode exists against this complaint and has been well proved in practice. Susceptible goats should be given one dose of 30c potency per week for four weeks and repeated one month later.

# 10.  EXTERNAL PARASITES

These include blowflies, lice and ticks, and the conditions to which they give rise are normally dealt with by washes and dips of various kinds. They rarely give rise to internal disease except in the case of ticks.

Blowfly or maggot infestation is seen in the summer months when flies lay their eggs on any open wound or unclean wound around the tail or dock. The maggots which develop attack the tissue causing severe irritation and distress.

Lice also cause severe itching and are more likely to be a source of trouble in the winter months when they cause the skin to become greasy, denuded of hair and unhealthy looking.

Ticks become active in spring and autumn and attach themselves to any convenient part of the skin and after sucking blood they drop off and undergo their life-cycle. Apart from diseases which they transmit (e.g. Louping Ill) they are a source of anaemia in the affected animal and deaths have been known to occur in severe infestations. They are easily plucked off by means of a small pair of tweezers.

Homoeopathically these pests can all be dealt with by using a 1/10 dilution of **HYPERCAL** and bathing the affected parts. This will help tissues to heal quickly.

# First Aid Remedies

The numerous accidents which call for emergency first-aid are varied in nature. Many of them necessitate surgical interference e.g. fractures and need not detain us here, although even in this instance there are remedies which will aid the healing process.

## A. WOUNDS/LACERATIONS

Probably the most efficacious dressing to be applied in the case of open wounds is **HYPERCAL** used in a dilution of 1/10. This will quickly ease pain and promote rapid healing. It will also help to heal ulcerated areas which would otherwise be slow to heal. This remedy is also available as a skin cream.

Punctured wounds e.g. those caused by penetration of sharp objects such as nails or bites call for the use of the remedy **LEDUM** using a 6c potency three times daily for three days. This should be followed by **HYPERICUM** 1m daily for seven days. The use of these two remedies will help prevent complications arising.

If injuries are sustained which are manifested by bruising with no breaking of the skin the remedy **ARNICA** is indispensable. It should be used in 30c potency in such cases, three times daily for three days.

## B. HAEMORRHAGE

There are many useful remedies to consider in cases of bleeding from whatever cause. The main ones are as follows:

**1. ARNICA**  This is a good general remedy for various types of haemorrhage especially those associated with injury of any kind. The blood is bright red. Suggested potency 30c one dose three times daily for three days.

**2. IPECACUANHA**   This remedy is associated with lack of appetite and possibly bleeding from the nose. The slightest exertion brings on a flow of blood. Suggested potency 6c one three times daily for five days.

**3. MELILOTUS**   This remedy is associated more with clover poisoning when haemorrhage occurs from different sources. Muscular weakness is present. Suggested potency 6c one dose every two hours for five doses.

**4. MILLEFOLIUM**   This remedy is most useful for nose-bleeding and animals showing distress in breathing. Suggested potency 6c one every hour for six doses.

**5. PHOSPHORUS**   When there are numerous small haemorrhages on the skin and/or gums. It is frequently associated with the treatment of haemorrhage from the lungs. Suggested potency 6c one dose three times daily for five days.

In addition to these remedies others based on the snake venom products may also be needed, as all snake venom remedies have an affinity with the circulation except the cobra venom (**NAJA**) which relates to the central nervous system. Remedies such as **VIPERA, CROTALUS, BOTHROPS** and **LACHESIS** could all be indicated depending on overall symptoms displayed. Reference should be made to a Materia Medica for their individual characteristics to determine the correct one.


# SNAKE BITE

This unfortunate occurrence sometimes arises in summer during particularly hot weather when adders tend to come out from uncovered areas. Bites around the head and lower limbs are areas most at risk. If the animal is bitten on the throat severe oedema and swelling occur which affects breathing and swallowing. This could lead to a fatal outcome. Homoeopathic remedies will do much to limit the constitutional damage and these include the following:

**1. ACONITUM**   This remedy should be given at once as it helps allay fear and shock. Suggested potency 1m one dose every hour for three doses.

**2. LACHESIS**   If the area surrounding the bite becomes bluish or purple this remedy is indicated. It is especially useful in bites affecting the throat. Suggested potency 1m one dose every hour for four doses.

**3. VIPERA** This is the remedy of the common or yellow viper which is the one most commonly implicated in the U.K. Blood from the wound is bright red. Suggested potency 1m one dose every two hours for four doses.

**4. CROTALUS** The rattlesnake poison potentised is a powerful anti-haemorrhagic agent and will quickly arrest bleeding in those cases when the surrounding skin becomes yellowish and cold. Suggested potency 1m one dose every hour for four doses.

**5. BOTHROPS** This remedy prepared from the venom of the lanceolate viper is particularly useful in controlling bleeding arising from bites to the lower limbs which as stated above are particularly at risk. Suggested potency 200c three times daily for three days.

**FOOTNOTE** In addition to these remedies **LEDUM** could also be used in conjunction with them because of its affinity with bites in general.


# POISONINGS

Goats would appear to be more prone to poisoning by various substances than other animals. Treatment of poisoning in the context of homoeopathic medicine, apart from first aid measures, depends on the animal's response to the particular poisoning and the symptoms the animal displays.

Poisonings have been reported from time to time due to one or other of the following plants and chemicals:

**1. RHODODENDRON** This is probably the commonest plant poisoning encountered among goats. Symptoms include excess salivation, attempts to vomit and inappetance. One case in the author's experience showed a good response to the remedies **RHUS TOX** and **NUX VOMICA** both in 1m potency but this was because the particular symptoms displayed suggested these remedies. Other digestive remedies which might have a beneficial effect on a tissue or organ basis are **COLCHICUM** 30c and **COLOCYNTHIS** 1m.

**2. KALE or RAPE** This plant can cause haemolysis of red blood cells causing the urine to become red. Weakness and anaemia are attendant features. Remedies which might help are **CHINA** 6c given four times daily for three days and **CROTALUS** 1m twice daily for five days.

**3. PRUNUS** The dried leaves of this plant family can be a source of poisoning when the animal will display difficult breathing due to the haemoglobin in the red cells being interfered with by the toxin contained in the leaves. Acute poisonings of this sort may be beyond help but milder cases could well respond to the remedies **CARBO VEG** 200c, **AMMON CARBONICUM** 30c and **BELLADONNA** 200c.

**4. RAGWORT** This weed is a common source of poisoning. The liver is the principal organ affected, cirrhosis eventually developing. This in time interferes with normal digestion leading to various upsets such as inappetance and wasting. Abdominal fluid (ascites) develops. Jaundice may or may not be present. Useful remedies to consider are **CARDUUS MARIANUS** 30c, **LYCOPODIUM** 1m and **PHOSPHORUS** 200c all of which have a beneficial action on liver function. If jaundice is present the remedy **CHELIDONIUM** and/or **CHIONANTHUS** could be given.

**5. LEAD** Objects containing this metal are a common hazard to grazing animals which may lack certain minerals in their system causing them to lick at different objects. Signs of poisoning include severe head shaking or head pressing leading to staggering and incoordination. Convulsions could also occur. Remedies to consider are **STRAMONIUM** 200c when the animals tends to fall to the left: **CICUTA VIROSA** 30c when recumbency is seen with the head bent backwards or the neck curved in an S shape. **AGARICUS** presents a picture of severe incoordination and staggering with jump or erratic movements, and should be used in 200c potency. **BELLADONNA** may be needed in 1m potency if convulsions develop while **PLUMBUM (lead)** 200c could be used in conjunction with any of the foregoing. **SULFONAL** is another useful remedy where staggering to the right side or falling backwards occurs. A potency of 200c may be needed.

# *Worming*

Worming in the larger animal (ruminants and horses) is not as straightforward as it is in dogs and cats because of the frequency of handling involved in the dosing process. This, however, can be overcome if necessary by employing the chosen remedy in liquid form and giving it in feed over the requisite period of dosing. The main worming remedies to consider are **KAMALA, CHENO-PODIUM** and **GRANATUM** in low potency e.g. 3c.

5ml. of this potency should be added to feed daily for fourteen days and repeated after an interval of one month. This is not really practical where large numbers are concerned and the procedure should be reserved for small numbers of goats e.g. up to ten animals.

# Infertility and Irregularities of the Oestrus Cycle

Does come into season at certain times of the year only, a normal season covering the period from early autumn to the beginning of spring. Infertility may have its origin in ovarian dysfunction or in abnormalities of the uterus and/or fallopian tubes, and may be temporary or permanent. In the absence of pregnancy, the oestrus cycle appears every 19–21 days. The heat itself varies in duration from 15 hours up to 36 hours in some cases. A prolonged heat frequently denotes late ovulation and could be a reason for delayed conception.

Five stages are recognised in the oestrus cycle.

**1. PRO-OESTRUS**   This is the period of preparation in which the Graafian follicle is growing and leads to the accumulation of follicular fluid. This fluid contains a seroid–hormone–oestradiol which along with the other substances known as oestrol and oestriol constitutes oestrogen.

**2. OESTRUS**   This is the period of excitement or desire in which the ovary has matured along with the Graafian follicle. Signs exhibited by the doe include loud calling and tail swishing and a mucous discharge may be present. Does in heat are usually mounted by other goats.

**3. METOESTRUS**   The day after oestrus is completed usually leads to rupture of the follicle and expulsion of the ovum. The follicular cavity is filled by the embryonic corpus luteum. This body secretes progesterone the function of which is to prepare the lining of the uterus for implantation of the fertilised ovum. At the same time oestrogen is inhibited and maturation of other follicles suppressed. It also control mammary development.

**4. DIOESTRUS**   During this period the uterine walls

thicken and the uterine glands become active. if pregnancy supervenes this condition persists, but in the absence of pregnancy the corpus luteum is resorbed, the withdrawal of progresterone initiating a new oestrus cycle.

**5. ANOESTRUS**   This is a period of inactivity which may occur as sequel to dioestrus or instead of it. It normally persists for a period of about seven or eight weeks after parturition.

We can now review the main causes of infertility where we might reasonably expect homoeopathic medication to be of benefit. These may be summarised as follows.

  a) Temperamental Factors
  b) Abortion of foetus at an early stage
  c) Endocrine Dysfunction
  d) Infection of the Genital Tract

### a) TEMPERAMENTAL FACTORS
Refusal to mate is uncommon but when it does occur it is worth trying the remedy **SEPIA** giving a dose of the 200c potency once per week for three weeks.

### b) ABORTION OF FOETUS AT AN EARLY STAGE
Apart from specific abortions non–specific forms may also occur. Frequently these take the form of an early discharge and the owner may be under the impression that no conception has taken place, when the animal comes into season later on. The main remedy to consider is **VIBURNUM OPULIS** in 30c potency giving it weekly for four weeks at the beginning of the following mating. Other remedies which have been successfully used in this connection are **PULSATILLA** 30c and **CALCAREA PHOS** 30c giving either once weekly for three weeks depending on overall symptoms.

### c) ENDOCRINE DYSFUNCTION
In one or other of its manifestations this is probably the most common breeding irregularity. Examples are sub-oestrus or silent heat, clinical features varying from absence of heat to does going several weeks or months without a definite oestrus period showing. Remedies to be considered in treatment include the following:

**1. SEPIA**   This should be given as a routine remedy

because of its overall effect on the ovaries and uterus. A potency of 200c once weekly for three weeks should suffice.

**2. PULSATILLA** This is a useful ovarian remedy sometimes associated with vaginal discharge of a creamy consistency. A potency of 30c should be used giving one dose per week for three weeks.

**3. PLATINA** This remedy also has a beneficial action on ovarian function. There may be catarrhal uterine discharge associated with urination, the urine having a reddish sediment. A potency of 30c should be tried daily for seven days.

**4. ALETRIS FARINOSA** The appetite is usually in abeyance if this remedy is indicated. There is a general uterine atony and a tendency to prolapse. Occasionally uterine bleeding takes place the blood being dark and membranous. A potency of 30c should be given twice weekly for four weeks.

**5. FOLLICULINUM** The intercurrent use of this nosode may aid the action of other remedies, using a potency of 30c daily for seven days.

### d) INFECTION OF THE GENITAL TRACT

# ANOESTRUS

From a study of the five stages of the oestrus cycle it will be seen that only one – anoestrus – is a departure from the normal state when it persists for longer than eight weeks after parturition. It is a fairly normal state of affairs. Remedies employed to initiate a new cycle include the following:

**1. PULSATILLA** This remedy should be employed in silent heat and is also useful after retained placenta. Suggested potency 200c one daily for five days.

**2. CALCAREA PHOS.** When indicated there is usually a profuse leucorrhoea, worse in the morning and sometimes accompanying a vaginitis. Suggested potency 30c one daily for five days, followed by one every second day for three doses.

**3. IODUM** This is a good remedy for lean does showing a harsh dry coat and excessive appetite together with an active temperament. Suggested potency 30c daily for ten days.

# CYSTIC OVARIES

Older does are more likely to be troubled with this condition than younger ones. The ovaries may contain several cysts and it is frequently associated with hyperplasia of the uterine endometrium. Clinical signs are those associated with irregular heat periods and nymphomania with possible changes in the shape of the pelvic girdle. For treatment the following remedies should be considered:

**1. APIS MEL.** This is a useful remedy for dissolving cysts by causing absorption of fluid. Suggested potency 6c twice daily for ten days.

**2. MUREX PURPUREA** This is a well tried remedy for excessive oestrus and for helping to regulate the oestrus cycle. Suggested potency 200c one dose per week for three weeks.

**3. NATRUM MURIATICUM** This remedy may be needed when there is an accompanying greenish vaginal discharge. The tissues involved are dry. Suggested potency 30c one daily for seven days.

**4. COLOCYNTHIS** When the condition is associated with abdominal pain causing the animal to stretch out with arched back. Suggested potency 1m daily for five days.

**5. PLATINA** Catarrhal vaginitis is usually present along with a reddish sediment in the urine. This is a good ovarian remedy in general especially for the less friendly doe. Suggested potency 30c twice daily for ten days.

**6. OOPHORINUM** This ovarian nosode frequently brings about resolution of the cysts if used in low potency e.g. 3x one dose three times daily for seven days.

# PERSISTENT CORPUS LUTEUM

By this term we mean the persistence of a functioning corpus luteum in the absence of pregnancy. It is usually associated with uterine changes, either pyometritis or endometrial hyperplasia. Remedies to be considered in alleviating the condition are as follows:

**1. FOLLICULINUM** The follicle hormone potentised will be found to be of service in promoting resolution. Suggested potency 30c daily for ten days.

**2. PULSATILLA** This remedy acts on the ovary helping to promote normal function. Suggested potency one daily for seven days.

**3. SEPIA** For regulating the function of the entire genital tract and aiding the action of other selected remedies. Suggested potency 200c one dose per week for two weeks.

# FREQUENT RETURN TO SERVICE

When this has its origin in endocrine dysfunction it is usually due to ovulating failure during an otherwise normal oestrus. It is a frequent cause of infertility. The following remedies will help promote ovulation.

**1. SEPIA** Suggested potency 200c once weekly for three weeks.

**2. PULSATILLA** There may be an accompanying vaginal discharge of semi-purulent material. Suggested potency 30c one dose three times weekly for three weeks.

**3. CALCAREA PHOS.** This is a useful remedy for the younger doe. Catarrhal vaginitis may be present. Suggested potency 30c one dose three times weekly for three weeks.

**4. OOPHORINUM** This ovarian nosode can be used in conjunction with any of the above. Suggested potency 30c daily for seven days.

# PREGNANCY

The gestation period for the average doe is around five months. Two remedies are important to consider for the maintenance of a healthy pregnancy, viz:

**1. VIBURNUM OPULIS** This is a proven remedy for use in the early stages of pregnancy e.g. up to one month or six weeks. It will help eliminate the tendency to early miscarriage of a non-specific nature and should be given in 30c potency three times per week for four weeks.

**2. CAULOPHYLLUM** This second remedy for use in the later stages has a long history of success in maintaining a healthy pregnancy. Not only will it help ensure a trouble-free parturition but will tone up the uterus generally and help expel lochia and placenta easily. It should be used in 30c potency three times per week for the last four weeks. If the second stage of labour is delayed or weak this remedy will take the place of the conventional pituitrin injection and speed up normal contractions.

The use of the remedy **ARNICA** 30c is advisable both at the time of kidding and also post-partum, one dose three times daily for two days should suffice. If by any chance the kidding is severe and prolonged the remedy **BELLIS PERENNIS** in 30c potency three times daily for two days will aid the action of Arnica.

# PROBLEMS ASSOCIATED WITH PREGNANCY

**1. ABORTION**   Apart from the non-specific abortion due to hormone imbalance and which is discussed under infertility there are a number of specific diseases associated with loss of foetus.
Chief among these are:
*CHLAMYDIA SPP* associated with enzootic abortion
*TOXOPLASMA* and *MYCOPLASMA* infection
*LISTERIOSIS* and *SALMONELLOSIS*
The specific abortions due to *BRUCELLA SPP (ABORTUS and MELITENSIS)* are much less likely to be a source of trouble in goats in the U.K. Indeed Br. melitensis while widespread in other countries does not fortunately affect goats in the U.K.

The homoeopathic approach to control of specific abortions lies in the use of the appropriate nosode. Once the particular organism has been identified it is a simple matter to have the nosode prepared and protection can then be provided on a flock basis (see section on vaccination procedure).

The abortions associated with the above organisms have been dealt with in the chapter on specific diseases.

# CLOUD BURST OR PSEUDO PREGNANCY

This is a hormonal disturbance due to the presence in the blood of the ovarian hormone progesterone. The doe appears to be pregnant and around the time when normal parturition would occur large quantities of fluid are expelled from the uterus, followed by the appearance of milk in the udder. This can be a troublesome condition and can last quite a long time. If a doe has experienced this particular problem in the past an attempt should be made to prevent it recurring. The following remedies may prove helpful:

**1. SEPIA 200c** One dose per week for three weeks should be given.

**2. PULSATILLA 30c** One dose per day for seven days followed by one dose of 200c per week for four weeks.

Together these two remedies should be sufficient for most cases but other remedies such as **PLATINA, PALLADIUM** and **CAULOPHYLLUM** may be needed. These remedies outlined should be given prior to normal service to susceptible animals.

Treatment as such once the condition has been established will be determined by the particular symptoms displayed but *SEPIA, APIS* and the nosode *OOPHERINUM* should cover the majority of uncomplicated cases.

# PROBLEMS ARISING POST-PARTUM

These are numerous and vary in severity but fortunately homoeopathy has a wide range of remedies available to meet the needs of most non-surgical conditions. These include haemorrhage, retained placenta, prolapse, metritis and milk fever.

**1. HAEMORRHAGE** Fortunately serious loss of blood at parturition is not common but should it occur the following remedies will help depending on the nature and type of bleeding e.g. if the blood accumulates in the uterus and is then expelled in a bright red flood the remedy **IPECACUANHA** is indicated using a 6c potency every hour for five doses. If the blood comes away as a steady drip, the remedy **CROTALUS** may be needed using a 1m potency every hour for four doses. Dark blood indicating venous origin may require the remedy **HAMAMELIS** while very dark stringy blood indicates the remedy **SECALE**. These last mentioned remedies should be used in 30c potency one dose every two hours for five doses.

Other proven remedies for the control of haemorrhage are **ARNICA, FICUS, MELILOTUS, MILLEFOLIUM** and **PHOSPHORUS** given according to overall symptoms presented.

# RETAINED PLACENTA

As in sheep and cattle goats have a cotyledonary placenta, the retention of which is not serious under normal circumstances. Remedies which have proved valuable in expelling retained membranes include **SEPIA** 30c, **PULSATILLA** 6c and **PYROGEN** 1m the first two given every hour for four doses and the last given in the same way. Retention of membranes after abortion and associated with blood-stained discharges may benefit more from the remedy **SABINA** using a 6c potency every hour for four doses.

# PUERPERAL METRITIS

This condition is an inflammation of the uterine endometrium associated with parturition and resulting in systemic involvement which can lead to illness of varying degrees of severity.

During the puerperium the lining of the uterus is commonly the seat of bacterial invasion. Any condition which delays the course of uterine involution tends to favour the onset of such infection e.g. difficult labour and/or retained placenta.

## CLINICAL SIGNS
An initial rise of temperature is followed by loss of appetite and general malaise. Respirations are increased and recumbency is usual. The pulse is either weak and thready or full and tense. The expression denotes anxiety. Acute metritis may involve the peritoneum, the inflammatory process being felt as a board-like mass on palpation of the abdomen. The vulva and vagina may be inflamed and dark red. Discharge is not always present but if it is it may vary from a yellowish colour through to blood-stained.

## TREATMENT
The following remedies should be considered:
**1. ACONITUM** The earlier this remedy is given the

more likely it is that a successful outcome will ensure. It is particularly indicated in those cases which arise with sudden intensity. The action helps allay shock and reduces fear and anxiety. Suggested potency 1m one dose every hour for four doses.

**2. BELLADONNA**  This is a good remedy to consider when there is a full bounding pulse, hot skin and dilated pupils accompanying a rise in temperature. There may be central nervous system involvement such as hyperexcitability. Suggested potency 1m one dose every hour for five doses.

**3. PYROGEN**  This artificial nosode is particularly indicated when a weak thready pulse alternates with a high temperature or vice versa. It is probably the most useful remedy in septic conditions where these conditions are present. Suggested potency 1m one dose every two hours for four doses.

**4. ECHINACEA**  The symptoms calling for this remedy are somewhat similar to the previous remedy except that with this particular remedy the temperature remains high. Suggested potency 6c one dose every hour for six doses.

**5. SABINA**  This is a useful remedy when the condition is associated with retention of afterbirth or miscarriage especially those cases showing blood-stained discharges. Suggested potency 6c one dose every hour for six doses.

**6. SECALE**  Somewhat similar in its indications to the previous remedy but discharges are dark and the blood is stringy and membranous. Suggested potency 30c twice daily for ten days.

**7. LACHESIS**  If the condition manifests itself in a haemorrhagic form with bluish or purple discolouration of surrounding parts and swelling of hind limbs this remedy should prove helpful. The throat is often swollen leading to difficulty in swallowing. Suggested potency 30c three times daily for five days.

# Rearing of Young Kids

When kids are weaned they should be given a course of the remedy **CALC PHOSPH** using a potency of 30c. One dose twice weekly for eight weeks and then reducing to one per week for another eight weeks will lay the foundation of good strong bone and tendon and enable the young kid to develop into a stronger adult. This will be reflected economically by the doe giving more and better quality milk. The first few months of the kid's life are the most important as what happens then will determine for good or ill much of its later life. Apart from the specific remedy mentioned above kids should be subjected to a programme of preventive medicine based on the use of nosodes against the commoner diseases.

# Materia Medica

**ABIES CANADENSIS. Hemlock Spruce.**
**N.O. Coniferae.**
The Ø is made from the fresh bark and young buds.

This plant has an affinity for mucous membranes generally and that of the stomach in particular, producing a catarrhal gastritis. Impairment of liver function occurs leading to flatulence and deficient bile-flow. Appetite is increased and hunger may be ravenous. It is chiefly used as a digestive remedy.

**ABROTANUM. Southernwood. N.O. Compositae.**
Tincture of fresh leaves.

This plant produces wasting of muscles of lower limbs and is used for animals showing this weakness. A prominent guiding symptom in the young animal is umbilical oozing of fluid. It is one of the remedies used to control worm infestation in young animals and also has a reputation in certain forms of acute arthritis where overall symptoms agree.

**ABSINTHIUM. Wormwood.**
Infusions of active principle.

The effect on the system of this substance is to produce a picture of confusion and convulsions preceded by trembling of muscles. There is a marked action on the central nervous system causing the patient to fall backwards. The pupils of the eye may show unequal dilation. It is one of the main remedies used in practice to control epileptiform seizures and fits of varying kinds.

**ACIDUM SALICYLICUM. Salicylic Acid.**
Trituration of powder.

This acid has an action on joints producing swellings and in some cases caries of bone. Gastric symptoms e.g.

bleeding are also prominent in its provings. Homoeopathically indicated in the treatment of rheumatic and osteo-arthritic conditions and idiopathic gastric bleeding.

## ACONITUM NAPELLUS. Monkshood.
### N.O. Ranunculaceae.
In the preparation of the Ø the entire plant is used as all parts contain aconitine the active principle.

This plant has an affinity for serous membranes and muscular tissues leading to functional disturbances. There is sudden involvement and tension in all parts. This remedy should be used in the early stages of all feverish conditions where there is sudden appearance of symptoms which may also show an aggravation when any extreme of temperature takes place. Predisposing factors which may produce a drug picture calling for **ACONITUM** include shock, operation and exposure to cold dry winds, or dry heat. It could be of use in puerperal conditions showing sudden involvement with peritoneal complications.

## ACTAEA RACEMOSA. Black Snake Root. Also referred to as Cimicifuga Racemosa. N.O. Ranunculaceae.
Trituration of its resin.

This plant resin has a wide range of action on various body systems, chief among which are the female genital and the articular leading to disturbances of the uterus in particular and small joint arthritis. Muscular pains are evident, affection of cervical vertebrae is evidenced by stiffening of neck muscles.

## ADONIS VERNALIS. Pheasant's Eye. N.O. Ranunculaceae.
Infusion of fresh plant.

The main action of the remedy which concerns us in veterinary practice is its cardial action which becomes weak leading to dropsy and scanty output of urine. It is one of the main remedies used in valvular disease and difficult respiration dependent on pulmonary congestion.

## AESCULUS HIPPOCASTANUM. Horse Chestnut.
### N.O. Sapindaceae.
The Ø is prepared from the fruit with capsule.

The main affinity of this plant is with the lower bowel

producing a state of venous congestion. There is a general
slowing down of the digestive and circulatory systems, the
liver and portal action becoming sluggish. This is associated with a tendency to dry stools. It is a useful remedy in
hepatic conditions with venous congestion affecting the
general circulation and it also has a place in the treatment
of congestive chest conditions.

## AGARICUS MUSCARIUS. Fly Agaric. N.O. Fungi.
The Ø is prepared from the fresh fungus.

Muscarin is the best known toxic compound of several
which are found in this fungus. Symptoms of poisoning
are generally delayed for anything up to twelve hours after
ingestion. The main sphere of action is on the central
nervous system producing a state of vertigo and delirium
followed by sleepiness. There are four recognised stages of
cerebral excitement. viz: 1. Slight stimulation. 2. Intoxica-
tion with mental excitement accompanied by twitching. 3.
Delirium. 4. Depression with soporific tendency. These
actions determine its use in certain conditions affecting the
central nervous system, e.g. cerebrocortical necrosis and
meningitis, which may accompany severe attacks of
hyomagnesaemia. Tympanitic conditions with flatus may
respond favourably while it also has a place as a rheumatic
remedy and in the treatment of some forms of muscular
cramp.

## AGNUS CASTUS. Chaste Tree. N.O. Verbenaceae.
Tincture of ripe berries.

One of the principal spheres of action relating to this
plant is the sexual system where it produces a lowering or
depression of functions with accompanying debility. In
the male there may be induration and swelling of testicles
and in the female sterility has been reported.

## ALETRIS FARINOSA. Star Grass.
## N.O. Haemodoraceae.
The Ø is prepared from the root.

This plant has an affinity with the female genital tract,
especially the uterus and is used mainly as an anti-abortion
remedy and in the treatment of uterine discharges and also
in silent heat in animals which may show an accompanying loss of appetite.

### ALLIUM CEPA. Onion. N.O. Liliaceae.
The Ø is prepared from the whole plant.

A picture of coryza with acrid nasal discharge and symptoms of laryngeal discomfort is associated with this plant. It could be indicated in the early stages of most catarrhal conditions producing the typical coryza.

### ALOE. Socotrine Aloes. N.O. Liliaceae
The Ø is prepared from a solution in spirit of the gum. Where disease and drug symptoms are confused this remedy is useful in restoring physiological balance. It should be considered in the treatment of bowel conditions with straining and passing of jelly-like stools containing mucus.

### ALUMEN. Potash Alum.
Trituration of the pure crystals.

Indicated in conditions affecting mucous membranes of various body systems, producing dryness: affections of the central nervous system are also common, resulting in varying degrees of paralysis.

### AMMONIUM CARBONICUM.
### Ammonium Carbonate.
This salt is used as a solution in distilled water from which the potencies are prepared.

It is primarily used in respiratory affections especially when there is an accompanying swelling of associated lymph glands. Emphysema, pulmonary oedema and fog fever are thoracic conditions which may be helped by this remedy. It is also useful in digestive upsets and may promote rumenal activity in sluggish states.

### AMMONIUM CAUSTICUM. Hydrate of Ammonia.
Potencies are again prepared from a solution in distilled water.

This salt has a similar but more pronounced action on mucous membranes to that of the carbonate producing ulcerations on these surfaces. It is also a powerful cardiac stimulant. Mucosal disease may call for its use; also respiratory conditions showing severe involvement of the lungs. There is usually an excess of mucus with moist cough when this remedy is indicated.

## ANGUSTURA VERA. N.O. *Rutaceae.*
Trituration of tree bark.

Bones and muscles come prominently into consideration when this plant is specified. Stiffness and limb pains of varying degree are prominent along with exostosis. Mild paralysis of legs has been noted. The action on bones may lead on to caries with possible fractures developing.

## ANTHRACINUM.
The Ø is prepared from affected tissue or culture dissolved in alcohol.

This nosode is indicated in the treatment of eruptive skin diseases which are characterised by boil-like swellings. Cellular tissue becomes indurated and swelling of associated lymph glands takes place. The characteristic lesion assumes the form of a hard swelling with a necrotic centre and surrounded by a blackened rim. It has proved useful in the treatment of septic bites.

## ANTIMONIUM ARSENICOSUM.
### Arseniate of Antimony.
Potencies are prepared from trituration of the dried salt dissolved in distilled water or alcohol.

This salt possesses a selective action on the lungs especially the upper left area and is used mainly in the treatment of emphysema and long-standing pneumonias. Coughing, if present, is worse on eating and the animal prefers to stand rather than lie down.

## ANTIMONIUM CRUDUM. Sulphide of Antimony.
Potencies prepared from trituration of the dried salt.

This substance exerts a strong influence on the stomach and skin producing conditions which are aggravated by heat. Any vesicular skin condition should be influenced favourably.

## ANTIMONIUM TARTARICUM. Tartar Emetic.
Trituration of the dried salt is the source of potencies.

Respiratory symptoms predominate with this drug, affections being accompanied by the production of excess mucus, although expectoration is difficult. The main action being on the respiratory system, we should expect this remedy to be beneficial in conditions such as bronchopneumonia and pulmonary oedema. Ailments requiring this remedy frequently show an accompanying drowsiness and lack of thirst. In pneumonic states the edges of the eyes may be covered with mucus.

## APIS MELLIFICA. The Honey Bee.
The Ø is prepared from the entire insect and also from the venom diluted with alcohol.

The poison of the bee acts on cellular tissue causing oedema and swelling. The production of oedema anywhere in the system may lead to a variety of acute and chronic conditions. Considering the well documented evidence of its sphere of action affecting all tissues and mucous membranes, we should consider this remedy in conditions showing oedematous swellings. Synovial swellings of joints may respond to its use and it has proved of value as an accessory remedy in the treatment of joint-ill in calves if given early. Respiratory conditions showing an excess of pulmonary fluid or oedema, e.g. fog fever, have been treated successfully with this remedy, while it has also been used to good effect in the treatment of cystic ovaries. All ailments are aggravated by heat and are thirstless.

## APOCYNUM CANNABINUM. Indian Hemp.
## N.O. Apocynaceae.
Infusions of the fresh plant.

This substance produces disturbance of gastric function along with affection of heart muscle leading to a slowing of its action. There is also a marked action on the uro-genetal system producing diuresis and uterine bleeding. The patient requiring this remedy may present symptoms of drowsiness or stupor. Upper respiratory symptoms are common e.g. nasal secretions of yellowish mucus.

## APOMORPHINUM.
This is one of the alkaloids of morphine and has a profound action on the vomiting centre of the brain producing several emissions preceded by increased secretion of saliva and mucus. Pupils become dilated. It is used in veterinary practice to produce complete emptying of stomach contents after suspected poisoning or ingestion of foreign matter, and homoeopathically to control prolonged and severe vomiting.

## *ARGENTUM NITRICUM. Silver Nitrate.*

This remedy is prepared by trituration of the salt and subsequent dissolving in alcohol or distilled water.

It produces incoordination of movement causing trembling in various parts. It has an irritant effect on mucous membranes producing a free-flowing muco-purulent discharge. Red blood cells are affected, anaemia being caused by their destruction. Its sphere of action makes it a useful remedy in eye conditions.

## *ARNICA MONTANA. Leopard's Bane.*
## *N.O. Compositae.*

The Ø is prepared from the whole fresh plant.

The action of this plant upon the system is practically synonymous with a state resulting from injuries or blows. It is known as the 'Fall Herb' and is used mainly for wounds and injuries where the skin remains unbroken. It has a marked affinity with blood-vessels leading to dilation, stasis and increased permeability. Thus various types of haemorrhage can occur. It reduces shock when given in potency and should be given routinely before and after surgical interference when it will also help control bleeding. Given after parturition it will hasten recovery of bruised tissue, while given during pregnancy at regular intervals, it will help promote normal easy parturition.

## *ARSENICUM ALBUM. Arsenic Trioxide.*

This remedy is prepared by trituration and subsequent dilution.

It is a deep-acting remedy and acts on every tissue of the body and its characteristic and definite symptoms make its use certain in many ailments. Discharges are acrid and burning and symptoms are relieved by heat. It is of use in many skin conditions associated with dryness, scaliness and itching. Coli-bacillosis and coccidiosis are conditions which may call for its use. It could also have a role to play in some forms of pneumonia when the patient may show a desire for small quantities of water and symptoms become worse towards midnight.

## *ARSENICUM IODATUM. Iodide of Arsenic.*

Potencies are prepared from the triturated salt dissolved in distilled water.

When discharges are persistently irritating and corro-

sive, this remedy may prove more beneficial than
**ARSEN. ALB.** The mucous membranes become red,
swollen and oedematous, especially in the respiratory
sphere. This remedy is frequently called for in bronchial
and pneumonic conditions which are at the convalescent
stage or in those ailments which have not responded
satisfactorily to seemingly indicated remedies.

### ASAFOETIDA. N.O. Umbelliferae

Ø obtained from gum resin and remedy potentised from
tincture this remedy should be remembered for its ability
to aid conditions associated with indigestion and flatulence
along with disorders of lactation; either excess or deficiency of milk.

### ATROPINUM. An Alkaloid of Belladonna.

This alkaloid produces some of the effects of Belladonna
itself but acts more particularly on the eyes causing
dilation of pupils: mucous membranes become extremely
dry. It could be indicated where overall symptoms of
Belladonna are not well-defined.

### BACILLINUM

This is one of the TB nosodes and in veterinary practice
has proved useful in the control of ringworm and similar
skin desquamations of a similar nature.

### BAPTISIA TINCTORIA. Wild Indigo.
### N.O. Leguminosae.

The Ø is prepared from fresh root and bark.

The symptoms produced by this plant relate mainly to
septicaemic conditions producing prostration and weakness. Low grade fevers and great muscular lethargy are
present in the symptomatology. All secretions and discharges are very offensive. Profuse salivation occurs
together with ulceration of gums which become discoloured. Tonsils and throat are dark red and stools tend to be
dysenteric.

### BARYTA CARBONICA. Barium Carbonate.

Potencies are prepared from trituration of the salt dissolved in distilled water.

The action of this salt produces symptoms and conditions more usually seen in old and very young subjects and

should be remembered as a useful remedy for certain conditions affecting the respiratory system especially.

## BARYTA MURIATICA. *Barium Chloride.*
Solution of salt in distilled water.

This salt produces periodic attacks of convulsions with spastic involvement of limbs. Ear discharges appear which are offensive and the parotid salivary glands become swollen. Induration of abdominal glands develops including the pancreas. It is indicated in many instances of ear canker and also in animals which show a tendency to develop glandular swellings along with the characteristic involvement of the nervous system.

## BELLADONNA. *Deadly Nightshade.*
## N.O. *Solanaceae.*
The Ø is prepared from the whole plant at flowering.

This plant produces a profound action on every part of the central nervous system causing a state of excitement and active congestion. The effect also on the skin, glands and vascular system is constant and specific. One of the main guiding symptoms in prescribing is the presence of a full bounding pulse in any feverish condition which may or may not accompany excitable states. Another guiding symptom is dilation of pupils.

## BELLIS PERENNIS. *Daisy. N.O. Compositae.*
The Ø is prepared from the whole fresh plant.

The main action of this little flower is on the muscular tissues of blood vessels producing a state of venous congestion. Systemic muscles become heavy, leading to a halting type of gait suggestive of pain. This is a useful remedy to aid recovery of tissues injured during cutting or after operation. Sprains and bruises in general come within its sphere of action and it should be kept in mind as an adjunct remedy along with **ARNICA**. Given post-partum it will hasten resolution of bruised tissue and enable the pelvic area to recover tone in a very short time.

## BENZOICUM ACIDUM. *Benzoic Acid.*
Potencies are prepared from gum benzoin which is triturated and dissolved in alcohol.

The most outstanding feature of this remedy relates to the urinary system producing changes in the colour and odour of the urine, which becomes dark red and aromatic with uric acid deposits. It may have a place in the treatment of some kidney and bladder conditions.

## BERBERIS VULGARIS. *Barberry.*
## N.O. *Berberidaceae.*
The Ø is prepared from the bark of the root.

This shrub of wide distribution has an affinity with most tissues. Symptoms which it produces are liable to alternate violently, e.g. feverish conditions with thirst can quickly give way to prostration without any desire for water. It acts forcibly on the venous system producing especially pelvic engorgements. The chief ailments which come within its sphere of action are those connected with liver and kidney leading to catarrhal inflammation of bile ducts and kidney pelvis. Jaundice frequently attends such conditions. Haematuria and cystitis may occur. In all these conditions there is an accompanying sacral weakness and tenderness over the loins.

## BERYLLIUM. *The Metal.*
Trituration and subsequent dissolving in alcohol produces the tincture from which the potencies are prepared.

This remedy is used mainly in respiratory conditions where the leading symptom is difficult breathing on slight exertion and which is out of proportion to clinical findings. Coughing and emphysema are usually present. This is a useful remedy in virus pneumonia, both acute and chronic forms, where symptoms are few while the animal is resting, but become pronounced on movement. It is a deep acting remedy and should not be used below 30c potency.

## BORAX. *Sodium Biborate.*
Potencies are prepared from trituration of the salt dissolved in distilled water.

This salt produces gastro-intestinal irritation with mouth symptoms of salivation and ulceration. With most complaints there is fear of downward motion. The specific action of this substance on the epithelium of the mouth, tongue and buccal mucosa determines its use as a remedy which will control such conditions as vesicular stomatitis and allied diseases, e.g. mucosal disease.

## BOTHROPS LANCIOLATUS. *Yellow Viper.*

Potencies are prepared from solution of the venom in glycerine.

This poison is associated with haemorrhages and subsequent rapid coagulation of blood. Septic involvement takes place as a rule and this is, therefore, a useful remedy in septic states showing haemorrhagic tendencies. Gangrenous conditions of the skin may respond to it.

## BROMIUM. *Bromine. The Element.*

Potencies are prepared from solutions in distilled water.

Bromine is found in combinations with iodine in the ash when seaweed is burned, and also in sea water. It acts chiefly on the mucous membrane of the respiratory tract, especially the upper trachea causing laryngeal spasm. This is a useful remedy for croup-like cough accompanied by rattling of mucus. Its indication in respiratory ailments is related to symptoms being aggravated on inspiration. It may be of use also in those conditions which arise from over-exposure to heat.

## BRYONIA ALBA. *White Bryony. Wild Hop.*
## N.O. *Cucurbitaceae.*

The Ø is prepared from the root before flowering takes place.

This important plant produces a glucoside which is capable of bringing on severe purgation. The plant itself exerts its main action on epithelial tissues and serous and synovial membranes. Some mucous surfaces are also affected producing an inflammatory response resulting in a fibrinous or serous exudate. This in turn leads to dryness of the affected tissue with later effusions into synovial cavities. Movement of the parts is interfered with and this leads to one of the main indications for its use, viz. all symptoms are worse from movement, the animal preferring to lie still. Pressure over affected areas relieves symptoms. This remedy may be extremely useful in treating the many respiratory conditions met with, especially pleurisy where the above symptom picture is seen.

## BUFO. *The Toad. N.O. Buforidae. Solution of Poison.*

This remedy is used in states of cerebral excitement sometimes severe enough to precipitate epilepsy. Dropsical states also develop. Has also been used in cases of exaggerated sexual impulses especially in the male.

### CACTUS GRANDIFLORUS. Night-blooming Cereus. N.O. Cactaceae.

The Ø is prepared from young stems and flowers.

The active principle of this plant acts on circular muscle fibres and has a marked affinity for the cardio-vascular system. It is mainly confined to the treatment of valvular disease, but it may also be of service in some conditions showing a haemorrhagic tendency.

### CALCAREA CARBONICA. Carbonate of Lime.

Trituration of the salt in alcohol or weak acid produces the solution from which potencies are prepared. The crude substance is found in the middle layer of the oyster shell.

This calcareous substance produces a lack of tone and muscular weakness with muscle spasm affecting both voluntary and involuntary muscles. Calcium is excreted quickly from the system and the intake of calcium salts does not ensure against conditions which may need the element prepared in the homoeopathic manner. **CALC. CARB.** is a strong constitutional remedy causing impaired nutrition, and animals which need potentised calcium show a tendency to eat strange objects. It is of value in the treatment of skeletal disorders of young animals and in the older animal suffering from osteomalacia.

### CALCAREA FLUORICA. Fluorspar.
### Fluoride of Lime.

Potencies are prepared from trituration of the salt with subsequent dilution in distilled water.

Crystals of this substance are found in the Haversian canals of bone. This increases the hardness, but in excess produces brittleness. It also occurs in tooth enamel and in the epidermis of the skin. Affinity with all these tissues may lead to the establishment of exostoses and glandular enlargements. It is in addition a powerful vascular remedy. The special sphere of action of this remedy lies in its relation to bone lesions especially exostoses. Both actinomycosis and actinobacillosis may benefit from its use.

### CALCAREA IODATA. Iodide of Lime.

Solution of salt in distilled water.

This remedy is used in cases of hardening of tissue,

especially glands and tonsils. The thyroid gland is also affected.

## CALCAREA PHOSPHORICA. *Phosphate of Lime.*
Potencies are prepared by adding dilute phosphoric acid to lime water, with trituration and subsequent dilution.

This salt has an affinity with tissues which are concerned with growth and the repair of cells. Assimilation may be difficult because of impaired nutrition and delayed development. Brittleness of bone is a common feature. This is a remedy of special value in the treatment of musculo-skeletal disorders of young stock.

## CALC. RENALIS PHOS *and*
## CALC. RENALIS URIC.
These two salts are indicated in cases of lithiasis due to the presence of stones of the respective substances. They aid the action of remedies such as **BERBERIS** and **HYDRANGEA** and Thlaspi and can be used along with them.

## CALENDULA OFFICINALIS. *Marigold.*
### N.O. Compositae.
The Ø is prepared from leaves and flowers.

Applied locally to open wounds and indolent ulcers this remedy will be found to be one of the most reliable healing agents we have. It will rapidly bring about resolution of tissue promoting healthy granulation. It should be used as a 1/10 dilution in warm water. It is helpful in treating contused wounds of the eyes and it can be combined with **HYPERICUM** when treating open wounds involving damage to nerves.

## CALICI VIRUS.
The potentised virus can be used either by itself or combined with other viruses in the treatment of gingivitis and respiratory conditions where it is thought that the disease is implicated.

## CAMPHORA. *Camphor. N.O. Lauraceae.*
Potencies are prepared from a solution of the gum in rectified spirit.

This substance produces a state of collapse with weakness and failing pulse. There is icy coldness of the entire body. It has a marked relationship to muscles and fasciae.

Certain forms of scour will benefit from this remedy, viz. those forms accompanied by collapse and extreme coldness of body surfaces. Any form of enteritis showing exhaustion and collapse may require this remedy. It may be needed in disease caused by salmonella species.

## CANNABIS SATIVA. American Hemp.
## N.O. Cannabinaceae.

The Ø is prepared from the flowering tops of the plant. This plant affects particularly the urinary, sexual and respiratory systems, conditions being accompanied by great fatigue. There is a tendency to pneumonia, pericarditis and retention of urine: which may lead to cystitis and a mucoid blood-stained urine.

## CANTHARIS. Spanish Fly.

The Ø is prepared by trituration of the insect with subsequent dilution in alcohol.

The poisonous substances contained in this insect attack particularly the urinary and sexual organs setting up violent inflammation. The skin is also markedly affected, a severe vesicular rash developing with intense itching. This is a valuable remedy in nephritis and cystitis typified by frequent attempts at urination, the urine itself containing blood as a rule. It may be indicated in certain post-partum inflammations and burning vesicular eczemas.

## CARBO VEGETABILIS. Vegetable Charcoal.

Potencies are prepared by trituration and subsequent dilution in alcohol.

Various tissues of the body have a marked affinity with this substance. The circulatory system is particularly affected leading to lack of oxygenation with a corresponding increase of carbon dioxide in the blood and tissues. This in turn leads to a lack of resistance to infections and to haemorrhages of dark blood which does not readily coagulate. Coldness of the body surface supervenes. When potentised this is a very useful remedy in all cases of collapse. Pulmonary congestions will benefit and it restores warmth and strength in cases of circulatory weakness. It acts more on the venous than on the arterial circulation. It could prove useful in some forms of rumenal stasis and bloat resulting from a sluggish portal circulation.

## CARDUUS MARIANUS. St. Mary's Thistle.
### N.O. Compositae.

Trituration of seeds dissolved in spirits.

This remedy is indicated in disorders arising from inefficiency of liver function. The action of the liver indicates its main use in veterinary practice. Cirrhotic conditions with accompanying dropsy respond well.

## CAULOPHYLLUM. Blue Cohosh.
### N.O. Berberidaceae.

The Ø is prepared from trituration of the root dissolved in alcohol.

This plant produces pathological states related to the female genital system. Extraordinary rigidity of the *os uteri* is set up leading to difficultes at parturition. Early abortions may occur due to uterine debility. These may be accopmpanied by fever and thirst. There is a tendency to retention of afterbirth with possible bleeding from the uterus. In potentised form this remedy will revive labour pains and could be used as an alternative to pituitrin injections once the os is open. It will be found useful in ringwomb and also in cases of uterine twist or displacement. In these cases it should be given frequently for three or four doses, e.g. hourly intervals. In animals which have had previous miscarriages it will help in establishing a normal pregnancy while post-partum it is one of the remedies to be considered for retained afterbirth.

## CAUSTICUM. Potassium Hydroxide.

This substance is prepared by the distillation of a mixture of equal parts of slaked lime and potassium bisulphate.

The main affinity is with the neuro-muscular system producing weakness and paresis of both types of muscle. Symptoms are aggravated by going from a cold atmosphere to a warm one. It may be of use in bronchitic conditions of older animals and in those which develop small sessile warts. it appears to have an antidotal effect in cases of lead poisoning and could be used in this connection as an adjunct to versenate injections.

## CEONOTHUS AMERICANUS. New Jersey Tea.
### N.O. Rhamnaceae.

Tincture of fresh leaves.

Splenic conditions in general come within the range of this remedy. Tenderness of the spleen may be evident. In the female, whitish vaginal discharges may arise. Chiefly used for conditions where it is thought that the spleen is involved.

## CHELIDONIUM. *Greater Celandine.*
## N.O. *Papaveraceae.*
The Ø is prepared from the whole plant, fresh at the time of flowering.

A specific action on the liver is produced by this plant. There is general lethargy and indisposition. The tongue is usually coated a dirty yellow and signs of jaundice may be seen in other visible mucous membranes. The liver is constantly upset with the production of clay-coloured stools. Because of its marked hepatic action it should be remembered when dealing with disturbances associated with a sluggish liver action. It may be of use in photosensitisation if signs of jaundice occur.

## CHIMAPHILLA UMBELLATA. *Ground Holly.*
## N.O. *Ericaceae.*
The Ø is prepared from the fresh plant.

The active principle of this plant produces a marked action on the kidneys and genital system of both sexes. In the eyes cataracts may develop. The urine is mucoid and blood-stained. Enlargement of prostate gland may develop while in the female mammary tumours and atrophy have both been recorded.

## CHININUM SULPHURICUM. *Sulphate of Quinine.*
Trituration of salt dissolved in alcohol.

This salt closely resembles the action of **CHINA** and should be remembered as a useful remedy in cases of debility due to loss of essential fluids. It affects the ear producing pain over the area and excessive secretion of wax. Conditions calling for its use tend to recur after apparent or real remissions.

## CHIONANTHUS VIRGINIA. *Fringe Tree.*
Tincture of bark.

This remedy is indicated in sluggish states of the liver including early cases of cirrhosis, accompanying a generalised loss of condition and in extreme cases emaciation. The stools produced are clay-coloured and there may be jaundice and high-coloured urine.

## CHLAMYDIA
This potentised nosode is used to prevent chlamydial infection in young does (see main text) and also in the treatment of kids showing the typical symptoms of gummy eyes and other manifestations.

## CICUTA VIROSA. *Water Hemlock.*
## N.O. *Umbelliferae.*
The Ø is prepared from the fresh root at the time of flowering.

The central nervous system is principally affected by this plant, spasmodic affections occurring. A characteristic feature is the head and neck twisted to one side accompanied by violence of one kind or another. Aggravation occurs from jarring or sudden movement. The general balance becomes upset and there is a tendency to fall to one side while the head and spine bend backwards. Various conditions of the brain and spinal cord may benefit from this remedy, e.g. cerebro-cortical necrosis, louping-ill and milk fever showing the typical lateral deviation of neck.

## CINCHONA OFFICINALIS. *China Officinalis.*
## *Peruvian Bark. N.O. Rubiaceae.*
The Ø is prepared from the dried bark dissolved in alcohol.

This plant is commonly referred to as 'China' and is the source of quinine. Large doses tend to produce toxic changes, e.g. nervous sensitivity, impaired leucocyte formation, haemorrhages, fever and diarrhoea. Weakness ensues from loss of body fluids. This remedy should be considered when an animal is suffering from debility or exhaustion after fluid loss, e.g. severe diarrhoea or haemorrhage. It is seldom indicated in the earlier stages of acute disease.

## CINERARIA MARITIMA. *Dusty Miller.*
## N.O. *Compositae.*
The Ø is prepared from the whole fresh plant.

The active principle is used mainly as an external application in eye conditions. The Ø should be diluted 1/10.

## CINNABARIS. *Mercuric Sulphide.*
Trituration of salt dissolved in alcohol.

The action of this substance relates mainly to the genito-urinary sphere where conditions such as albuminuria and balanitis tend to occur. Warts develop in the inguinal area. Eye conditions are also common such as blepharitis and ophthalmia with purulent discharge. Sometimes the ear is affected producing a dry itching condition with scurf around the pinna. Chiefly used in practice where other mercurial remedies have given less than satisfactory results.

## COBALTUM. *The Metal.*
## COBALTUM CHLORIDUM. *The Salt.*
Both these remedies are used mainly in the 30c potency in the treatment of cobalt deficiency and give good results over a period of a few weeks.

## COCCULUS. *Indian Cockle. N.O. Menispermacrae.*
The Ø is prepared from powdered seeds which contain an alkaloid pectoxin.

The active principle produces spasmodic and paretic affections deriving from the CNS (Cerebrum), not the spinal cord. There is a strong tendency to vomit due to the action on the vomiting centre which appears to be dependent on movement. Mainly used in travel sickness where symptoms agree.

## COCCUS CACTI. *Cochineal.*
The Ø is prepared from the dried bodies of the female insects.

This substance has an affinity for mucous membranes producing catarrhal inflammation. Viscid mucus accumulates in the air passages leading to difficulty in expectoration and spasmodic coughing. Dysuria is common, the urine being scanty and leaving a reddish deposit on standing. It is mainly used in affections of the respiratory and urinary systems.

## COLCHICUM AUTUMNALE. *Meadow Saffron. N.O. Liliaceae.*
The Ø is prepared from the bulb.

This plant affects muscular tissues, periosteum and synovial membranes of joints. It also possesses an antiallergic and anti-inflammatory action which interferes with the natural recuperative powers of the body. Illnesses which may require this remedy are usually acute and severe, accompanied frequently by effusions in the small joints. It has a particular value in the treatment of rumenal bloat when it may have to be repeated at frequent intervals. Autumnal diarrhoea and dysentery also may be helped, the latter accompanied by tympany and tenesmus. One of its guiding symptoms is aversion to food, while complaints requiring it are generally worse from movement.

## COLOCYNTHIS. *Bitter Cucumber.*
### *N.O. Cucurbitaceae.*
The Ø is prepared from the fruit and contains a glucoside – colocynthin.

This plant is purgative and causes violent inflammatory lesions of the gastro-intestinal tract. Both onset of and relief fropm symptoms are abrupt. Diarrhoea is yellowish and forcibly expelled. Relief is obtained by movement while aggravation occurs after eating or drinking.

## CONDURANGO. *Condor Plant.*
The Ø is prepared from bark in tincture.

This plant produces a glucoside-condurangin, which affects the nervous system causing an exaggerated gait. It can act constitutionally in promoting the general well-being of the patient. More specifically there is an action on epithelial tissue causing hardening which may lead on to tumour formation. A guiding symptom is said to be cracks at the corners of the mouth. Chiefly used as a remedy to combat incipient cancerous states especially those in the abdomen.

## CONIUM MACULATUM. *Hemlock.*
### *N.O. Umbelliferae.*
The Ø is prepared from the fresh plant.

The alkaloid of this plant produces a paralytic action on nerve ganglia, especially the motor nerve endings. This leads to stiffness and a paralysis which tends to travel forward or upward. This remedy is of importance in treating paraplegic conditions and any weakness of hind limbs.

## CONVALLARIA MAJALIS. Lily of the Valley. N.O. Liliaceae.

The Ø is prepared from the fresh plant.

The active principle has the power to increase the quality of the heart's action and this determines its main use as a remedy in congestive heart conditions. It has little action on the heart muscle and is used mainly in valvular disease.

## COPAIVA. Balsam of Peru. N.O. Leguminosae.

The Ø is prepared from the balsam.

This substance produces a marked action on mucous membranes, especially those of the urinary and respiratory tracts causing a catarrhal inflammation. This action makes the remedy useful in the treatment of urethritis and cystitis. Pyelonephritis is one of the commoner conditions which could be helped.

## CORTISONE

The potentised steroid is used in practice to combat the effects of the over prescribing of the crude substance where very often a single dose of the 200c potency will suffice along with clearing remedies such as **NUX VOMICA** and **THUJA.** In lower potency e.g. 12c–30c it helps in certain skin conditions where dryness and redness predominate along with excessive itching.

## CRATAEGUS. Hawthorn. N.O. Rosaceae.

The Ø is prepared from the ripe fruit.

The active principle produces a fall in blood pressure and brings on dyspnoea. It acts on the heart muscle causing an increase in the number and quality of contractions. The specific action on the heart muscle makes this a particularly useful remedy in the treatment of arrhythmic heart conditions.

## CROTALUS HORRIDUS. Rattlesnake.

The Ø is prepared from trituration of the venom with lactose and subsequent dilution in glycerine.

This venom produces sepsis, haemorrhages and jaundice with decomposition of blood. The marked action of this poison on the vascular system makes it a valuable remedy in the treatment of many low-grade septic states with circulatory involvement, e.g. puerperal fever and wound infections. Septic conditions are accompanied by oozing of blood from any body orifice and are usually attended by jaundice. It should help in conditions such as adder-bite and clover poisoning.

### CROTON TIGLIUM. *Croton Oil Seeds.*
### N.O. *Euphorbiaceae.*
The Ø is prepared from the oil obtained from the seeds.

This oil produces violent diarrhoea and skin eruptions causing inflammation with a tendency to vesicle formation. This is one of the many useful remedies for controlling diarrhoea. This is usually accompanied by great urging, the stool being watery.

### CRYPTOCOCCUS
This potentised nosode is used as for chlamaydia and calici and can be combined with them if need be in multiple infections.

### CUBEBA OFFICINALIS. *Cubebs. N.O. Piperaceae.*
The Ø is prepared from the dried unripe fruit.

The active principle acts on mucous membranes producing a catarrhal inflammation. Those of the uro-genital tract are particularly affected, the urine becoming cloudy and albuminous.

### CUPRUM ACETICUM. *Copper Acetate.*
Potencies are prepared from a solution in distilled water.

This salt produces cramping of muscles, spasms and paralytic conditions. It is used chiefly in the treatment of copper deficiency, especially when accompanied by muscle cramping or stiffness. The arsenate of copper and the metal itself are similarly used.

### CUPRUM METALLICUM. *Metallic Copper.*
The Ø is prepared from trituration of the metal.

The symptoms produced by this metal are characterised by violence including paroxysms of cramping pains which follow no particular pattern. Muscles become contracted and show twitchings. In the central nervous system fits and convulsions occur and may take an epileptiform nature. The head is drawn to one side.

### CURARE, *Woorari. Arrow Poison.*
The Ø is prepared from dilutions in alcohol.

This poison produces muscular paralysis without impairing sensation or consciousness. Reflex action is diminished and a state of motor paralysis sets in. It decreases the output of adrenalin and brings about a state of nervous debility.

### DAMIANA
The active principle of this plant has an affinity for the sexual system and is used mainly to promote libido in the male animal where sexual drive is weak. The action and results are variable but it is a remedy to keep in mind in this connection.

### DIGITALIS PURPUREA. *Foxglove.*
### N.O. *Scrophulariaceae.*
The Ø is prepared from the leaves.

The active principle of the foxglove causes marked slowness of the heart's action, the pulse being weak and irregular. This is a commonly used remedy in heart conditions helping to regulate the beat and producing a stable pulse. By increasing the output of the heart when used in low potencies it aids valvular function. This in turn increases the output of urine and helps reduce oedema.

### DROSERA ROTUNDIFOLIA. *Sundew.*
### N.O. *Droseraceae.*
The Ø is prepared from the fresh plant.

The lymphatic and pleural systems together with synovial membranes are all affected by this plant. The laryngeal area is also subject to inflammatory processes, any stimulus producing a hypersensitive reaction.

### DULCAMARA. *Woody Nightshade.* N.O. *Solanaceae.*
The Ø is prepared from the green stems and leaves before flowering.

This plant belongs to the same family as **BELLADONNA, HYOSCYAMUS** and **STRAMONIUM**. Tissue affinites are with mucous membranes, glands and kidneys, producing inflammatory changes and interstitial haemorrhages. This remedy may benefit those conditions which arise as a result of exposure to wet and cold, especially when damp evenings follow a warm day. Such conditions commonly occur in autumn and diarrhoea occurring then may benefit. It has proved useful in the treatment of ringworm and could have a beneficial action on large fleshy warts.

### ECHINACEA ANGUSTIFOLIA. *Rudbeckia.* N.O. *Compositae.*
The Ø is prepared from the whole plant.

Acute toxaemias with septic involvement of various tissues come within the sphere of action of this plant. It is a valuable remedy in the treatment of post-partum puerperal conditions where sepsis is evident. Generalised septic states having their origin in infected bites or stings will also benefit. This remedy acts best in low decimal potencies.

### E. COLI
This organism is found in the bowel and plays an essential role in the digestive process. As a remedy the nosode is used in bowel conditions where scouring develops after stress in the young animal or where the balance of the bowel flora has been interfered with.

### EEL SERUM.
The Ø is prepared from dried serum or solution in distilled water.

The serum of the eel produces an action on the blood equivalent to toxaemia. It affects the kidney particularly with secondary effects on the liver. Renal deposits are found in the urine along with haemoglobin. Threatened anaemic states develop. The cardiac system is also affected, sudden fainting spells being common.

### EPIGEA REPENS. *Trailing Arbutus. N.O. Ericaceae.*
The Ø is prepared from tincture of fresh leaves.

The main action of this remedy is on the urinary system where it produces a state of strangury with the production of renal calculi. It should be remembered in this connection as a useful remedy in the treatment of urethral and bladder stones.

### EUPHRASIA OFFICINALIS. *Eyebright.* N.O. *Scrophulariaceae.*
The Ø is prepared from the whole plant.

The active principle acts mainly on the conjunctival mucous membrane producing lachrymation. The cornea is also affected, opacities being common. This is one of the most useful remedies in the treatment of a variety of eye conditions, principally conjunctivitis and corneal ulcerations. Internal treatment should be supplemented by its use externally as a lotion diluted 1/10.

### F.V.R. Nosode.
This is the potentised virus prepared from a case of feline viral rhinotracheitis. It can be used in both the prophylactic and therapeutic manner, and in the former combined with other viral nosodes.

### FERRUM IODATUM. Iodide of Iron.
Potencies are prepared from trituration of crystals subsequently dissolved in alcohol.

This salt is chiefly of interest as a remedy for iron deficiency associated with respiratory distress, mucous discharges containing blood being present. Metallic iron (Ferrum Metallicum) and Chloride of Iron (Ferrum Muriaticum) are also used in the treatment of iron deficiency, the former particularly for younger animals and the latter more indicated when heart symptoms such as weak thready pulse are present.

### FERRUM PHOSPHORICUM. Ferric Phosphate.
Potencies are prepared from a solution in distilled water.

Febrile conditions in general are associated with this salt. It is frequently used in the early stages of inflammatory conditions which develop less rapidly than those calling for **ACONITUM**. Throat involvement is often the key to its selection. Pulmonary congestions may call for its use if haemorrhages are also present.

### FICUS RELIGIOSA. Pakur. N.O. Moraceae.
The Ø is prepared from fresh leaves in alcohol.

Haemorrhages of various kinds are associated with the toxic effects of this plant. Any condition which produces bleeding of a bright red character may indicate the need for this remedy. It could be of value in Coccidiosis, but generally respiratory rather than digestive upsets determine its use.

## FLOR DE PIEDRA. *also known as* LOPHOPHYTUM

The Ø is prepared from the root of the plant after trituration and extraction in alcohol.

This remedy has an affinity with the thyroid gland causing functional changes. It has proved useful in liver insufficiency and mild forms of pancreatitis.

## FLUORICUM ACIDUM. *Hydrofluoric Acid.*

Potencies are prepared by distilling calcium fluoride with sulphuric acid.

It has an action on most tissues producing deep-seated ulcers and lesions of a destructive nature. It has been used successfully in the treatment of Actinomycosis and in ulcerative conditions of the mouth and throat. Any necrotic condition of bone is likely to benefit.

## FOLLICULINUM.

This is one of the ovarian hormones which has a beneficial action on the skin. Used mainly in practice in cases of miliary eczema and alopecia of both sexes. It can also be used in the treatment of eczemas of non-hormonal origin where the typical purply rashes predominate.

## FORMICA. *Formic Acid. The Ant.*
### N.O. *Hymenoptera.*

Tincture made from live ants. This acid produces rheumatic-like pains along with deposits in the small joints. Occasionally in severe cases the spinal cord may be affected giving rise to a state of temporary paralysis. It is chiefly used in veterinary practice as an anti-arthritis remedy especially affecting carpal and tarsal areas.

## GAERTNER-BACH

Marked emaciation or malnutrition is associated with this nosode. Chronic gastro-enteritis occurs and there is a tendency for the animal to become infested with worms. There is an inability to digest fat. Chiefly used in the young animal showing malnutrition associated with other digestive problems.

## GALEGA OFFICINALIS. *Goat's Rue.*
### N.O. *Leguminosae*

Ø prepared from tincture of whole plant.

This remedy has proved useful in controlling excess lactation. It also has a reputation for increasing the appetite.

## GELSEMIUM SEMPERVIRENS. Yellow Jasmine. N.O. Loganiaceae.
The Ø is prepared from the bark of the root.

The affinity of this plant is with the nervous system producing varying degrees of motor paralysis. This remedy has proved helpful as a supportive measure in hypomagnesaemia, aiding restoring of normal movement. Single paralysis of different nerves, e.g. the radial may also benefit. Conditions which call for its use are usually attended by weakness and muscle tremors.

## GLONOINUM. Nitro-Glycerine.
Potencies are prepared from dilutions in alcohol.

This substance has an affinity with the brain and circulatory system causing sudden and violent convulsions and also congestion in the arterial system leading to throbbing and pulsations, seen in superficial vessels. it will be found of use in brain conditions arising from over-exposure to heat or the effects of the sun. It may also help the convulsions associated with hypomagnesaemia and allied conditions.

## GRAPHITES. Black Lead.
Potencies are prepared from triturations dissolved in alcohol.

This form of carbon has an affinity with sklin and hooves. Eruptions are common and its action on connective tissue tends to produce fibrotic conditions associated with malnutrition. Loss of hair occurs while purply moist eruptions ooze a sticky discharge. Abrasions develop into ulcers which may suppurate. Favourable sites for eczema are in the bends of joints and behind the ears.

## GUNPOWDER
This a mixture of carbon, sulphur and the nitrate of potassium. It has proved useful in the treatment of abscesses and deep-seated septic cellulitis. It should be considered also as an additional remedy alongside those others which relate to blood-poisoning.

## HAMAMELIS VIRGINICA. *Witch Hazel.*
### N.O. *Hamamelidaceae.*
The Ø is prepared from fresh bark of twigs and roots.

This plant has an affinity with the venous circulation producing congestions and haemorrhages. The action on the veins is one of relaxation, with consequent engorgement. Any condition showing venous engorgement or congestion with passive haemorrhage should show improvement from the use of this remedy.

## HECLA LAVA. *Hecla.*
Potencies are prepared from trituration of the volcanic ash. Present in this ash are the substances which accompany lava formation, viz. Alumina, Lime and Silica.

Lymphoid tissue and the skeleton are areas which show the greatest affinity for this substance. The remedy is useful in the treatment of exostoses or tumours of the facial bones and in caries arising from dental disease. It has proved successful in the treatment of actinomycosis affecting the maxillary and mandibular bones. It should help in the treatment of bony tumours generally.

## HELLEBORUS NIGER. *Christmas Rose.*
### N.O. *Ranunculaceae.*
The Ø is produced from the juice of the fresh root.

The affinity of this plant is with the central nervous system and the alimentary canal. The kidneys are involved to a lesser extent. Vertigo-like movements arise together with convulsions. Vomiting and purging take place, stools being dysenteric. Heart action is slowed.

## HEPAR SULPHURIS CALCAREUM.
### *Impure Calcium Sulphide.*
This substance is prepared by burning crude calcium carbonate with flowers of sulphur. Potencies are then prepared from the triturated ash.

This remedy is associated with suppurative processes producing conditions which are extremely sensitive to touch. It causes catarrhal and purulent inflammation of the mucous membranes of the respiratory and alimentary tracts with involvement of the skin and lymphatic system. This remedy has a wide range of action and should be considered in any suppurative process showing extreme sensitivity to touch indicating acute pain, e.g. acute summer mastitis. Low potencies of this remedy promote suppuration while high potencies – 200c and upwards – may abort the purulent process and promote resolution.

## HIPPOZAENIUM
This nosode has been known for a long time having been made from glanders, a notifiable equine disease no longer encountered in Britain. It has a wide range of use in many catarrhal conditions which are characterised by glutinous or honey-coloured discharges, e.g. sinusitis and ozaena with or without ulceration of nasal cartilages. It could be of great benefit in some forms of chronic viral rhinitis.

## HYDRANGEA ARBORESCONS.
### N.O. Hydrangeaceae.
The Ø is prepared from fresh leaves and young shoots.

This plant exerts a strong influence on the urinary system, especially on the bladder where it helps dissolve gravel. The prostate gland also comes within its range of action.

## HYDRASTIS CANADENSIS. Golden Seal.
### N.O. Ranunculaceae.
The Ø is prepared from the fresh root.

Mucous membranes are affected by this plant, a catarrhal inflammation being established. Secretions generally are thick and yellow. Any catarrhal condition resulting in a muco-purulent discharge will come within the scope of this remedy, e.g. mild forms of metritis or sinusitis.

## HYDROCOTYLE ASIATICA. Indian Pennywort.
### N.O. Umbelliferae.
The Ø is prepared from the whole plant.

The main difficulty of this plant is with the skin and female genital system. It also has a lesser effect on the action of the liver. Skin conditions showing thickening of epidermis and roughening come within its sphere of action.

## HYOSCYAMUS NIGER. Henbane. N.O. Solanaceae.
The Ø is prepared from the fresh plant.

The active principle disturbs the central nervous system producing symptoms of brain excitement and mania.

Conditions which call for its use are not accompanied by inflammation (cf. **BELLADONNA**).

## HYPERICUM PERFORATUM. St. John's Wort. N.O. Hypericaceae.

The Ø is prepared from the whole fresh plant.

The active principle is capable of causing sensitivity to light on some skins in the absence of melanin pigment. The main affinity is with the nervous system causing hypersensitivity. Sloughing and necrosis of skin may take place. This remedy is of prime importance in the treatment of lacerated wounds where nerve endings are damaged. In spinal injuries, especially of the coccygeal area, it gives good results. The specific action on nerves suggests its use in tetanus where, given early after injury, it helps prevent the spread of toxin. It can be used externally for lacerated wounds along with **CALENDULA**, both in a strength of 1/10. It has been found useful in the treatment of photosensitisation and similar allergies.

## IODUM. Iodine. The Element.

Potencies are prepared from the tincture prepared by dissolving the element in alcohol. A 1% tincture is the strength used in preparation.

In large doses – iodism – sinuses and eyes are at first involved leading to conjunctivitis and bronchitis. Iodine has a special affinity with the thyroid gland. Weakness and atrophy of muscles may follow excessive intake. The skin becomes dry and withered-looking and the appetite becomes voracious. Conditions which show a characteristic oppositeness of symptoms, e.g. tissue hyperplasia or atrophy may need this remedy. It may be of use in ovarian dysfunction when the ovaries appear small and shrunken on rectal examination. It is a useful gland remedy and its specific relation to the thyroid should not be forgotten.

## IPECACUANHA. N.O. Rubiacea.

The Ø is prepared from the dried root. Emetine, an alkaloid is its principal constituent.

This plant is associated with haemorrhages and has found a use in the treatment of post-partum bleeding where the blood comes in gushes. Some forms of white scour may also benefit, particularly those showing tenesmus with greenish stools.

## IRIS VERSICOLOUR. *Blue Flag, N.O. Iridaceae.*

The Ø is prepared from the fresh root.

This plant produces an action on various glands, principally the salivary, intestinal pancreas and thyroid. it has a reputation also for aiding the secretion of bile. Due to its action on the thyroid gland swelling of the throat may occur. The remedy is chiefly used in veterinary practice in the treatment of disorders of the pancreas where it has given consistently good results.

## KALI ARSENICUM. *Fowler's Solution.*
## *Potassium Arsenite.*

Dilutions of this salt provide the Ø.

The main action 'which concerns us in goat keeping is exerted on the skin, a dry scaly eczema with itching being established. It is a good general skin remedy.

## KALI BICHROMICUM. *Potassium Bichromate.*

Potencies are prepared from a solution in distilled water.

This salt acts on the mucous membranes of the stomach, intestines and respiratory tract with lesser involvement of other organs. Feverish states are absent. The action on the mucous membranes produces a catarrhal discharge of a tough stringy character with a yellow colour. This particular type of discharge is a strong guiding symptom for its use. It could be used in broncho-pneumonia, sinusitis and pyelonephritis.

## KALI CARBONICUM. *Potassium Carbonate.*

Potencies are prepared from a solution in distilled water.

This salt is found in all plants and in the soil, the colloid material of cells containing potassium.

It produces a generalised weakness which is common to other potassium salts. Feverish states are absent. It could be a useful convalescent remedy.

## KALI CHLORICUM. *Potassium Chlorate.*

Potencies are prepared from a solution in distilled water.

The urinary organs are chiefly affected, producing a blood-stained and albuminous urine with a high phosphate content.

## KALI HYDRIODICUM. *Potassium Iodide.*

Potencies are prepared from triturations dissolved in alcohol.

This important drug produces an acrid watery discharge from the eyes and also acts on fibrous and connective tissue. Glandular swellings also appear. This is a widely used remedy in various conditions showing the typical eye and respiratory symptoms.

### KREOSOTUM. *Beechwood Kreosote.*

The Ø is prepared from solution in rectified spirit.

This substance produces haemorrhages from small wounds with burning discharges and ulcerations. It also causes rapid decomposition of body fluids. Blepharitis occurs with a tendency to gangrene of the skin, while in the female dark blood appears from the uterus. This substance has been successfully used in threatened gangrenous states showing the typical early stages of spongy bleeding and ulceration.

### LACHESIS. *Bushmaster. Surucucu Snake.*

Trituration of venom dissolved in alcohol is the source of the solution which yields the potencies.

This venom produces decomposition of blood rendering it more fluid. There is a strong tendency to haemorrhage and sepsis with profound prostration. This is a useful remedy for Adder bites helping to prevent septic complications and reduced swelling. It is particularly valuable if the throat develops inflammation causing left-sided swelling which may involve the parotid gland. Where haemorrhage takes place the blood is dark and does not clot readily while the skin surrounding any lesion assumes a purplish appearance.

### LATHYRUS SATIVUS. *Chick Pea.*
### N.O. *Leguminosae.*

The Ø is prepared from the flower and the pods.

This plant affects the anterior columns of the spinal cord producing paralysis of the lower extremities. Nerve power generally is weakened. It should be considered in recumbent conditions associated with mineral deficiencies and in any state involving nerve weakness leading to local paralysis.

### LEDUM PALUSTRE. *Marsh tea. Wild Rosemary.*
### N.O. *Ericaceae.*

The Ø is prepared from the whole plant.

The active principle produces tetanus-like symptoms with twitching of muscles. It is one of the main remedies for punctured wounds, especially when the surrounding area becomes cold and discoloured. Insect bites respond well. Also injuries to the eye.

### LEMNA MINOR. Duckweed. N.O. Lemnaceae.
The Ø is prepared from whole fresh plants.

This is a remedy for catarrhal conditions affecting mainly the nasal passages; a muco-purulent nasal discharge develops which is extremely offensive. In the alimentary sphere diarrhoea and flatulence can occur.

### LILIUM TIGRINUM. Tiger Lily. N.O. Liliaceae.
The Ø is prepared from fresh leaves and flowers.

The action is mainly on the pelvic organs producing conditions which arise from uterine or ovarian disturbances. Urine is scanty and frequently passed. An irregular pulse accompanies an increased heart rate. Congestion and blood-stained discharges arise from the uterus and there may be slight prolapse. Indicated in some forms of pyometra where blood is present and also in ovarian disturbances.

### LITHIUM CARBONICUM. Lithium Carbonate.
The Ø is prepared from trituration of the dried salt.

This salt produces a chronic arthritic state with a uric acid diathesis. There is difficulty in passing urine which contains mucus and a red, sandy deposit. Cystitis develops leading to a dark urine. It is a useful remedy to consider in some forms of arthritis and urinary conditions producing uric acid deposits.

### LOBELIA INFLATA. Indian Tobacco.
### N.O. Lobeliceae.
The Ø is prepared from the dried leaves with subsequent dilution in alcohol.

The active principle acts as a vaso-motor stimulant impeding respiration and producing symptoms of inappetance and relaxation of muscles. It is of value in emphysematous conditions and as a general convalescent remedy.

## LYCOPLUS VIRGINICUS. *Bugle Weed.*
### N.O. *Labiatae.*
The Ø is prepared from fresh whole plant.

The active principle of this plant reduces blood pressure and causes passive haemorrhages. The main sphere of action which concerns veterinary practice is on the cardiac system where the pulse becomes weak and irregular. The heart's action is increased and is accompanied by difficult breathing and cyanosis. Breathing assumes a wheezy character and may produce a blood-tinged cough.

## LYCOPODIUM CLAVATUM. *Club Moss.*
### N.O. *Lycopodiaceae.*
The Ø is prepared from trituration of the spores and dilution in alcohol. The spores are inactive until triturated and potentised.

The active principle acts chiefly on the digestive and renal systems. The respiratory system is also affected, pneumonia being a frequent complication. There is general lack of gastric function and very little food will satisfy. The abdomen becomes bloated with tenderness over the liver. The glycogenic function of the liver is interfered with. This is a very useful remedy in various digestive urinary and respiratory conditions, a guiding symptom being that complaints frequently show an aggravation in the late afternoon or early evening. It is the first remedy of choice in the digestive form of acetonaemia while its action on the skin suggests its use in alopecia.

## MAGNESIA PHOSPHORICA.
### *Phosphate of Magnesium.*
Potencies are prepared from trituration of the salt in solution.

This salt acts on muscles producing a cramping effect with spasm. It is a valuable remedy to be remembered as supportive treatment in hypomagnesaemia where its prompt use will limit the tendency to brain damage and help fix the element in the system, as otherwise it may be quickly excreted.

## MALANDRINUM.
This nosode has been developed from the condition known as grease in the horse after trituration of affected material and discharge. It is used mainly in the treatment

of chronic skin eruptions and discharges. In this connection it is worth remembering as a remedy which might help some forms of ear canker.

### MEDUSA. *Jelly Fish.*
Ø prepared from the living animal and dissolved in alcohol.

This uncommon remedy is chiefly used to promote lactation after parturition: also in some forms of vesicular skin eruptions.

### MELILOTUS. *Sweet Clover. N.O. Leguminosae.*
The Ø is prepared from the whole fresh plant.

This plant is associated with profuse haemorrhages. Clover contains a haemolytic agent which prevents clotting of blood after mechanical injuries. This is more likely to happen if animals are fed mouldy hay. It should be remembered as a possibly useful remedy in haematomas and subcutaneous bleeding of unknown origin.

### MERCURIUS. *Mercurius Solubilis. Mercury.*
Potencies are prepared from triturations and dilutions in alcohol.

This metal affects most organs and tissues producing cellular degeneration with consequent anaemia. Salivation accompanies most complaints and gums become spongy and bleed easily. Diarrhoea is common, stools being slimy and blood-stained. Conditions calling for its use are worse in the period from sunset to sunrise.

### MERCURIUS CORROSIVUS. *Mercuric Chloride. Corrosive Sublimate.*
Potencies are prepared from triturations and subsequent dilution.

This salt has a somewhat similar action to **MERCURIUS SOL.**, but generally the symptoms produced are more severe. It produces severe tenesmus of the lower bowel leading to dysentery and also has a destructive action on kidney tissue. Discharges from mucous surfaces assume a greenish tinge. It could be of value in severe cases of Coccidiosis.

### MERCURIUS CYANATUS. *Cyanate of Mercury.*
Potencies are prepared from triturations and dilutions.

This particular salt produces an action similar to that

associated with bacterial toxins. A haemorrhagic tendency with prostration is a common feature. Ulceration of the mucous membranes of the mouth and throat commonly occur which suggests its use in kid diphtheria. A greyish membrane surrounds these ulcerated surfaces. The phyaryngeal area is one of the main regions to be affected, redness of the membrane preceding necrosis in the later stages.

### MERCURIUS DULCIS. Calomel. Mercurous Chloride.
Potencies are prepared from triturations and dilution.
This salt has an affinity with the ear and liver especially. Hepatitis with jaundice may result. It is worth considering as a possibly useful remedy in mild forms of cirrhosis.

### MERCURIUS IODATUS FLAVUS.
### Yellow Iodide of Mercury.
Potencies are prepared from triturations in dilution.
**MERCUROUS IODIDE FLAVUS** produces a tendency to glandular induration with attendant coating of the tongue. Sub-maxillary and parotid glands become swollen, more pronounced on the right side. Various swellings of glandular tissue come within the sphere of this remedy, e.g. parotitis and lymphadenitis generally. It could be of value in actinobacillosis when lesions attack on the right side.

### MERCURIUS IODATUS RUBER.
### Red Iodide of Mercury.
Potencies are prepared from trituration of the salt.
**MERCURIUS IODATUS RUBER** also has a tendency to produce glandular swellings, but in this case the left side of the throat is involved. Stiffness of neck muscles may be a prominent symptom.

### MILLEFOLIUM. Yarrow. N.O. Compositae.
The Ø is prepared from the whole plant.
Haemorrhages occur from various parts from the action of this plant. The blood is bright red.

### MINERAL EXTRACT.
This substance has recently been researched and has been shown to have a beneficial effect on certain forms of joint trouble, e.g. arthritis and stiffness especially of the carpal and tarsal areas.

## MIXED GRASSES.

Some animals show an allergic response to grasses in early spring and summer when excessive itching and skin lesions develop. A combination of various grasses in potency appear to help these conditions and can be combined with other selected remedies.

## MORGAN-BACH.

Clinical observation has revealed the symptom picture of the bacillus Morgan to cover in general digestive and respiratory conditions with a secondary action on fibrous tissues and skin used mainly in practice to treat inflammatory conditions especially acute eczema combined with appropriate remedies.

## MUREX PURPUREA. *Purple Fish.*

The Ø is prepared from the dried secretion of the purple gland of one of the Murex species.

It exerts its action mainly on the female genital system producing irregularities of the oestrus cycle. It has been employed both in anoestrus and for stimulating ovulation, but probably it will give best results in cystic ovary leading to nymphomania.

## MURIATICUM ACIDUM. *Hydrochloric Acid.*

Potencies are prepared from dilutions, in distilled water.

This acid produces a blood condition analogous to that associated with septic feverish states of a chronic nature. There is a tendency for ulcers to form. The throat becomes dark red and oedematous while ulceration of the lips accompanies swollen gums and neck glands.

## MYRISTICA SEBIFERA. N.O. *Myristicaceae*

Potencies prepared from trituration of the gum obtained from the bark.

This remedy is associated with septic conditions of small joints and superficial ulcerations. It is especially useful for treatment of suppurations around the coronary band. Superficial infection of the umbilicus in the new-born kid could also benefit from its use.

## NAJA TRIPUDIANS. *Cobra.*

Potencies are prepared from trituration of the venom and

subsequent dilution in alcohol. Alternatively the Ø may be prepared by dilution of the pure venom.

This poison produces a bulbar paralysis. Haemorrhages are scanty but oedema is marked. The underlying tissues appear dark purple after a bite, blood-stained fluid being present in large quantities. Loss of limb control supervenes. The heart is markedly affected. It could be of use in angio-neurotic oedema.

## NATRUM MURIATICUM. Common Salt. Sodium Chloride.

Potencies are prepared from triturations dissolved in distilled water.

Excessive intake of common salt leads to anaemia, evidenced by dropsy or oedema of various parts. White blood cells are increased while mucous membranes are rendered dry. This is a remedy which is of value in unthrifty conditions arising as a result of anaemia or chronic nephritis.

## NATRUM SULPHURICUM. Sodium Sulphate.

The Ø is prepared from trituration of the salt.

Glauber's Salts (as it is commonly called) produces a state of weakness where the animal has been exposed to damp. The liver is affected and there is a tendency to wart formation. Hepatitis sometimes occurs with jaundice. Flatulent distension and watery diarrhoea supervene. Experience has shown that this remedy has proved to be of great value where there has been a history of head injury leading to a variety of seemingly unrelated conditions.

## NITRICUM ACIDUM. Nitric Acid.

Potencies are prepared from a solution in distilled water.

This acid particularly affects body outlets where skin and mucous membranes meet. It produces ulceration and blisters in the mouth and causes offensive discharges. The ulceration may also affect mucous membranes elsewhere and it has been of benefit in some forms of mucosal disease in valves.

## NUX VOMICA. Poison Nut. N.O. Loganiaeceae.

The Ø is prepared from the seeds.

Digestive disturbances and congestions are associated

with this plant, flatulence and indigestion being commonly encountered. Stools are generally hard. Rumenal stasis is likely to benefit.

## OCIMUM CANUM. N.O. Labiatae.

The Ø is prepared from the fresh leaves.

This remedy exerts its action mainly on the urinary system producing a turbid urine of a deep yellow colour. The urine itself is slimy and purulent with a musky sweet smell. Mainly used in urinary disturbances showing the typical symptoms.

## OPIUM. Poppy. N.O. Papaveraceae.

The Ø is prepared from the powder after trituration.

Opium produces an insensibility of the nervous system with stupor and torpor. There is lack of vital reaction. All complaints are characterised by soporific states. Pupils are contracted and the eyes assume a staring look.

## OVARIUM.

This is also one of the ovarian hormones in potency. It covers a range of action similar to **FOLLICULINUM** but the results have been shown to be less satisfactory than with the latter remedy.

## PALLADIUM. The Metal.

Potencies are prepared from triturations and subsequent dilution in alcohol.

This element produces its main action on the female genital system, especially the ovaries causing inflammation with a tendency to pelvic peritonitis. The right ovary is more usually affected. Pelvic disorders arising as a result of ovaritis should also benefit.

## PANCREAS – Pancreatinum.

The Ø is prepared from pancreas extract after trituration.

It is used on various disorders of the pancreas either on its own or combined with selected remedies to suit the individual case. In pancreatitis it can be used along with the digestive enzyme Trypsin.

## PAREIRA. Velvet Leaf. N.O. Menispermaceae.

The Ø is prepared from tincture of fresh root.

The active principle of this plant exerts its action mainly

on the urinary system producing catarrhal inflammation of the bladder with a tendency to calculus formation. In the female there may be vaginal or uterine discharge. It is a useful remedy to consider in cases of vesical calculus where the animal is presented with acute strangury and distress.

## PAROTIDINUM.
This is the nosode of mumps and in veterinary practice it is a useful remedy in the treatment of cases of parotid gland swellings and associated structures. It may be used either on its own or combined with indicated remedies.

## PASTEURELLA.
This is a nosode prepared from cultures of the Pasteurella organism in cases of disease. It is usually potentised to 30c and used along with selected remedies in cases of pasteurellosis.

## PETROLEUM. *Rock Spirit.*
The Ø is prepared from the oil.

This substance produces cutaneous eruptions and catarrhal mucous membranes. Eczematous eruptions develop around ears and eyelids and feet producing fissures which are slow to heal. The skin is usually dry. Complaints are usually worse in cold weather. A useful remedy for some forms of chronic skin conditions where symptoms agree.

## PHOSPHORICUM ACIDUM. *Phosphoric Acid.*
Potencies are prepared from a dilution of the acid in distilled water.

This acid produces a debilitating state in which flatulence and diarrhoea are common features.

## PHOSPHORUS. *The Element.*
The Ø is prepared from trituration of red phosphorus.

This important substance produces an inflammatory and degenerative effect on mucous membranes and causes bone destruction and necrosis of liver and other parenchymatous organs. It has a profound effect on eye structures especially the retina and iris. There is a marked haemorrhagic diathesis associated with this remedy, and small haemorrhages appear on skin and mucous membranes. Its uses in practice are wide and varied and it is one of the most important remedies in the pharmacopoeia.

## PHYTOLACCA DECANDRA. Poke Root. N.O. Phytolaccaceae.

The Ø is prepared from the whole fresh plant.

A state of restlessness and prostration is associated with this plant, together with glandular swellings. It is chiefly used in veterinary practice to combat swellings of the mammary glands in particular when the glands become hard and painful. Abscesses may develop together with mastitis of varying degree. In the male testicular swelling may occur. The remedy is of immense value in mastitis and other forms of mammary swellings.

## PLUMBUM METALLICUM. The Metal or Lead.

The Ø is prepared from trituration with sugar of milk.

A state of paralysis preceded by pain is produced by exposure to or ingestion with lead. It affects the central nervous system and also causes liver damage leading to jaundiced states. Blood pictures show anaemia. Paralyses of lower limbs develop and convulsions are common leading to coma. It should be remembered as a useful remedy to consider in degenerative renal states associated with liver involvement.

## PODOPHYLLUM. May Apple. N.O. Ranuculaceae.

The Ø is prepared from the whole fresh plants.

The active principle of this plant exerts its action mainly on the duodenum and small intestine causing an enteritis. The liver and rectum are also affected. Distension of the abdomen occurs with a tendency to lie on the abdomen. Colicky pains develop with tenderness over the liver. A watery greenish diarrhoea may alternate with constipation. It is a useful remedy for gastro-intestinal disorders especially of young animals and for liver and peritoneal congestion.

## PSEUDOMONAS.

This is the potentised organism used in the treatment of cases of Pseudomonas infection. It can be combined with selected remedies in this event.

## PSORINUM. Scabies Vesicle.

The Ø is prepared from trituration of the dried vesicle.

This nosode produces a state of debility, especially after acute illness with skin symptoms predominating. All discharges are unpleasant. Chronic ophthalmia is occasionally seen along with otitis media and externa producing an offensive brownish discharge. Skin conditions are accompanied by severe itching. Animals needing this remedy prefer warmth.

## PTELEA. *Water Ash. N.O. Rutaceae.*
The Ø is prepared from the bark or root.

This plant produces its main action on the stomach and liver. Hepatitis occurs with tenderness over liver and stomach areas. This is a good 'cleansing' remedy in that it will aid elimination of toxins and thereby help clear conditions such as eczema and asthmatic tendencies.

## PULSATILLA. *Anemone. N.O. Ranunculaceae.*
The Ø is prepared from the entire plant when in flower.

Mucous membranes come within the sphere of action of this plant, thick muco-purulent discharges being produced. It has proved useful in the treatment of ovarian hypofunction and in retained placenta.

## PYROGENIUM. *Artificial Sepsin.*
The Ø is prepared from solutions of raw protein in distilled water.

This nosode has a specific relation to septic inflammations associated with offensive discharges. It is indicated in all septic conditions where the animal presents a clinical picture of raised temperature alternating with a weak thready pulse, or vice versa. It should be used in potencies of 200c and upwards.

## RANUNCULUS BULBOSUS. *Buttercup.*
## *N.O. Ranunculaceae.*
The Ø is prepared from the whole plant.

The action is mainly on muscular tissue and skin producing a hypersensitivity to touch. Skin lesions take the form of papular and vesicular eruptions which may cluster together into over-shaped groups.

## RESCUE REMEDY.
This is one of the many Bach Flower remedies and possibly the one most widely known and used. These remedies are not potentised like homoeopathic remedies but have been shown in practice to exert remarkable

curative properties. Rescue Remedy is used to benefit the patient after exposure to any traumatic experience e.g. stress, shock and post-operative trauma. A very useful remedy to revive weak kids after birth.

### RHEUM. Rhubarb. N.O. Polygonaceae
The Ø is prepared from trituration of the dried root distilled in alcohol.

This remedy is associated with bowel conditions producing a specific sour-smelling diarrhoea. Shivering and straining precede the onset of diarrhoea.

### RHODODENDRON. Snow Rose. N.O. Ericaceae.
The Ø is prepared from the fresh leaves.

This shrub is associated with muscular and joint stiffness. Orchitis is not uncommon with the testicles becoming hard and indurated.

### RHUS TOXICODENDRON. Poison Ivy. N.O. Anacardiaceae.
The Ø is prepared from the fresh leaves.

The active principles of this tree affect skin and muscles together with mucous membranes and fibrous tissues producing tearing pains and blistery eruptions. Symptoms of stiffness are relieved by movement. Involvement of the skin leads to a reddish rash with vesicles and produces a cellulitis of neighbouring tissues. It could be a useful remedy in muscle and joint conditions which show a characteristic improvement on exercise.

### RUMEX CRISPUS. Yellow Dock. N.O. Polygonaceae.
The Ø is prepared from the fresh root.

The active principle of this plant causes a diminution in the secretions from mucous membranes. Chronic gastritis occurs accompanied by an aversion to food and a watery diarrhoea. Mucous discharges take place from the trachea and nose. These tend to assume a frothy appearance. It is a useful remedy in some forms of respiratory affections.

### RUTA GRAVEOLENS. Rue. N.O. Rutaceae.
The Ø is prepared from the whole fresh plant.

Ruta produces its action on the periosteum and cartilages with a secondary effect on eyes and uterus. Deposits form particularly around the carpal joints. It also has a selective action on the lower bowel and rectum and could prove useful in mild forms of rectal prolapse. It has been known to facilitate labour by increasing the tone of uterine contractions.

### SABINA. Savine. N.O. Coniferae.
The Ø is prepared from the oil dissolved in alcohol.

The uterus is the main seat of action producing a tendency to abortion. There is also an action on fibrous tissues and serous membranes. It is associated with haemorrhages of bright red blood which remains fluid. This remedy has its main use in uterine conditions including retained placenta. Persistent post-partum bleeding may also be arrested.

### SANGUINARIA. Blood Root. N.O. Papaveraceae.
The Ø is prepared from the fresh root.

An alkaloid – sanguinarine – contained in this plant has an affinity with the circulatory system leading to congestion and redness of skin. The female genital system is affected, inflammation of ovaries occurring. Small cutaneous haemorrhages arise in various sites. Stiffness of forelegs, especially the left shoulder region may be seen.

### SECALE CORNUTUM. Ergot of Rye. N.O. Fungi.
The Ø is prepared from the fresh fungus.

Ergot produces marked contraction of smooth muscle causing a diminution of blood supply to various areas. This is particularly seen in peripheral blood vessels, especially of the feet. Stools are dark-green alternating with dysentery. Bleeding of dark blood occurs from the uterus with putrid discharges. The skin becomes dry and shrivelled-looking with a tendency for gangrene to form. Because of its circulatory action and its effect on smooth muscle it is useful in some uterine conditions, e.g. post-partum bleeding of dark blood and in any condition with impairment of peripheral circulation.

### SEPIA OFFICINALIS. Cuttlefish.
Potencies are prepared from trituration of the dried liquid from the ink bag.

Portal congestion and stasis are associated with this substance along with disturbances of function in the female genital system. Prolapse of uterus may occur or a tendency thereto. It will regulate the entire oestrus cycle and should always be given as a routine preliminary remedy in treatment. It also has an action on the skin and has given good results in the treatment of ringworm. Post-partum discharges of various sorts will usually respond. It is also capable of encouraging the natural maternal instinct in those animals which are indifferent or hostile to their offspring.

### SILICEA. *Pure Flint.*
Potencies are prepared from triturations dissolved in alcohol.

The main action of this substance is on bone where it is capable of causing caries and necrosis. It also causes abscesses and fistulate of connective tissue with secondary fibrous growths. There is a tendency for all wounds to suppurate. This is a widely used remedy indicated in many suppurative processes of a chronic nature. It gives good results in summer mastitis and will hasten resolution of the udder, by its ability to absorb scar tissue.

### SOLIDAGO VIRGA. *Golden Rod. N.O. Compositae.*
The Ø is prepared from the whole fresh plant.

This plant produces an inflammatory action on paren-chymatous organs, particularly the kidney. The urine is scanty, reddish and accompanied by albumen deposits. Prostatic enlargement is frequently encountered. It is a useful remedy to consider in certain cases of renal insufficiency either with or without prostatic enlargement in the male animal.

### SPIGELIA. *Pink Root. N.O. Logianaceae.*
The Ø is prepared from the dried herb.

This plant has an affinity for the nervous system and also exerts an action on the cardiac region and the eye, producing ophthalmia and dilated pupils. A useful remedy for certain eye conditions especially if pain above the eyes can be elicited from the patient.

### SPONGIA TOSTA. *Roasted Sponge.*
Potencies are prepared from dilutions in alcohol.

This substance produces symptoms related to the respiratory and cardiac spheres. The lymphatic system is also affected. The thyroid gland becomes enlarged. The general action on glands suggests its use in lymphadenitis. It is principally used as a heart remedy after respiratory infections.

### SQUILLA MARITIMA. Sea Onion. N.O. Liliaceae.
The Ø is prepared from the dried bulb.

This substance acts especially on the mucous membranes of the respiratory tract. The digestive and renal systems are also affected. Nasal discharges develop accompanied by a dry cough which later becomes mucoid. There is urging to urinate, the urine being watery and profuse. It is a useful remedy for heart and kidney affections being especially valuable in dropsical conditions.

### STAPHISAGRIA. Stavesacre. N.O. Ranunculaceae.
The Ø is prepared from the seeds.

The nervous system is mainly involved with this plant but there is also an action on the genito-urinary tract and the skin. A useful remedy in cystitis, but probably its most important indication is as a post-operative remedy where it acts on the mental level reducing psychological trauma and hastening the healing of wounds. It is also of benefit in the treatment of hormonal eczemas and alopecias.

### STRAMONIUM. Thorn Apple. N.O. Solanaceae.
The Ø is prepared from the whole fresh plant and fruit.

The active principle of this shrub produces its main action on the central nervous system, especially the cerebrum, producing a staggering gait with a tendency to fall forward on to the left side. Dilation of pupils occurs with a fixed staring look. A useful remedy to consider in brain disturbances where overall symptoms agree.

### STREPTOCOCCUS and STAPHYLOCOCCUS.
**STREPTOCOCCUS** nosode is used in conditions associated with infections by this organism, e.g. erythematous rashes, tonsillitis and nephritis with associated pyelitis. It can be combined with other selected remedies. **STAPHYLOCOCCUS AURENS** is the main remedy to consider in staphylococcal affections, e.g. abscesses and mastitis. These nosodes are usually used in 30c potency.

### STROPHANTHUS. Onage. N.O. Apocynaceae.
The Ø is prepared from the seeds dissolved in alcohol.

This shrub produces an increase in the contractile power of striped muscle. It acts especially on the heart increasing stystole. The amount of urine passed is increased and albuminuria may be present. This is a useful heart remedy to help remove oedema. It is a safe and useful diuretic especially for the older animal.

### STRYCHNINUM. Strychnine. Alkaloid contained in Nux Vomica.
Potencies are prepared from solutions in distilled water.

This alkaloid stimulates the motor centres of the spinal cord and increases the depth of respirations. All reflexes are rendered more active and pupils become dilated. Rigidity of muscles occurs especially of the neck and back with jerking and twitching of limbs. Muscle tremors and tetanic convulsions set in rapidly. This remedy may prove useful in severe forms of hypomagnesaemia or cerebro-cortical necrosis if the specific symptoms are present.

### SULFONAL. A derivative of Coal Tar.
The Ø is prepared from solution in alcohol or trituration with lactose.

This substance affects the central nervous system causing irregular movements, twitchings and incoordination of muscles which become stiff with a paralytic tendency. A useful remedy to consider in cases of cerebro-cortical affections showing the typical neuro-muscular symptoms.

### SULPHUR. The Element.
Potencies are prepared from trituration and subsequent dilution in alcohol.

This element has a wide range of action, but it is chiefly used in skin conditions such as mange and eczema and also as an inter-current remedy to aid the action of other remedies.

### SYMPHYTUM. Comfrey. N.O. Boraginaceae.
The Ø is prepared from the fresh plant.

The root of this plant produces a substance which stimulates growth of epithelium on ulcerated surfaces and hastens union of bone in fractures. It should always be given as a routine remedy in fractures as an aid to healing. Together with other vulneraries like **ARNICA** it is indicated in the treatment of injuries in general. It is also a prominent eye remedy.

## SYZYGIUM. *Jumbul. N.O. Myrtaceae.*
The Ø is prepared from trituration of seeds and subsequent dilution in alcohol.

This plant exerts an action on the pancreas and this its use in practice, especially in diabetes where it reduces the specific gravity of the urine and reduces thirst and controls output of urine.

## TABACUM. *Tobacco.*
This substance produces nausea and vomiting with intermittent pulse and weakness. In extreme cases there is a picture of muscular weakness and collapse.

Its main use in goat medicine would be in the treatment of sickness associated with movement.

## TARENTULA CUBENSIS. *Cuban Tarantula Spider.* N.O. *Araneida*
The Ø is prepared from trituration of the whole spider dissolved in alcohol.

This is another remedy to consider in the treatment of abscesses which are slow to heal and subject to sloughing of overlying skin. Such conditions are attended by pain and occasional pyrexia, which is worse late in the day. Systemic symptoms include prostration and diarrhoea.

## TARENTULA HISPANIA. *Spanish Spider.*
The Ø is prepared from trituration of the whole insect.

Hysterical states are associated with this poison, and there is also a stimulatory action on the uro-genital system. A useful remedy to consider in cases of hysteria and epilepsy accompanied or preceded by excitement. Excessive libido (satyriasis) in the male may be helped.

## TELLURIUM. *The Metal.*
The Ø is prepared from trituration with lactose.

This element exerts an influence on skin, eyes and ears. There is also an action on the sacral region. Cataracts and conjunctivitis develop. In the skin, herpetic eruptions appear which assume an annular shape. This remedy is a useful one to consider in some forms of ear trouble where eruptions appear on the ear flap.

## TEREBINTHINA. *Oil of Turpentine.*

Potencies are prepared from a solution in alcohol.

Haemorrhages are produced from various surfaces, urinary symptoms predominating. There is difficulty in urinating and blood commonly occurs n the urine. Bleeding may also take place in the uterus, especially after parturition. It is principally used in acute nephritis associated with haematuria and a sweet-smelling urine. This odour has been likened to that of violets. It also has a use in the treatment of gaseous bloat when low potencies will help.

## TESTOSTERONE.

This is a male hormone secreted by the testicle and is used mainly in the treatment of miliary eczema and alopecia in the castrated male. It has been shown clinically to be less effective in this connection than the female hormones **FOLLICULINUM** and **OVARIUM**. It has also been used with varying success in the treatment of anal adenoma.

## THALLIUM ACETAS.

The metallic salt is triturated and dissolved in alcohol.

This metal exerts an action on the endocrine system and also on the skin and neuro-muscular system where it produces paralysis followed by muscular atrophy. The skin conditions frequently result in alopecia. It is used mainly in the treatment of trophic skin conditions e.g. chronic alopecia and myelitis.

## THLASPI BURSA PASTORIS. *Shepherd's Purse.*
### N.O. *Cruciferae.*

The Ø is prepared from the fresh plant.

This plant produces haemorrhages with a uric acid diathesis. It favours expulsion of blood clots from the uterus and is indicated after miscarriage. There is frequency of urination, the urine being heavy and turbid with a reddish sediment. Cystitis is commonly seen with blood-stained urine.

## THUJA OCCIDENTALIS. *Arbor Vitae.*
### N.O. *Coniferae.*

The Ø is prepared from fresh twigs.

Thuja produces a condition which favours the formation of warty growths and tumours. It acts mainly on the skin and uro-genital system. Warts and herpetic eruptions develop, the neck and abdomen being the favourite sites. This remedy is of great importance in the treatment of skin conditions accompanied by the development of warty growths which bleed easily. Papillomatous warts are especially influenced and this action may be enhanced by the external application of the remedy in Ø form.

## THYROIDINUM. *Thyroid Gland.*
Potencies are prepared from triturations and dilution in alcohol.

Anaemia, emaciation and muscular weakness are associated with excess of thyroid secretion. There is dilation of pupils with prominence. Heart rate is increased. This remedy may be of use in the treatment of alopecia and allied skin conditions.

## TRINITROTOLUENE. *T.N.T.*
Potencies are prepared from a solution in distilled water.

This substance exerts a destructive influence on red blood cells causing haemolysis with consequent loss of haemoglobin. This produces anaemia and this is the principle of treatment by this remedy. It could be of use in babesiasis and similar conditions.

## TUBERCULINUM BOVINUM.
This nosode should be considered if a case of tuberculosis is encountered, but apart from this it is indicated in the treatment of osteomyelitis and some forms of peritonitis and pleurisy with effusions.

## URANIUM NITRICUM. *Uranium Nitrate.*
The Ø is prepared from solution in distilled water.

Glycosuria and polyuria are the main objective symptoms associated with the provings of this salt. There is a marked action on the pancreas where it influences digestive function. Large amounts of urine are passed. This is a useful remedy in pancreatitis where it follows well after the remedy **IRIS VERSICOLOR**.

## URTICA URENS. *Stinging Nettle. N.O. Urticaceae.*
The Ø is prepared from the fresh plant.

The nettle causes agalactia with a tendency to the formation of calculi. There is a general uric acid diathesis with urticarial swellings being present on the skin. There is diminished secretion of urine. The mammary glands become enlarged with surrounding oedema. This is a very useful remedy in various renal and skin conditions. In the treatment of uric acid tendencies it acts by thickening the urine which contains increased deposits of urates.

### USTILAGO MAYDIS. Corn Smut. N.O. Fungi.

The Ø is prepared from trituration of the fungus with lactose.

This substance has an affinity for the genital organs of both sexes, particularly the female where the uterus is markedly affected. Alopecia of varying degrees develops accompanying a dry coat. Uterine bleeding occurs, the blood being bright red and partly clotted. Haemorrhages occur post-partum. In the male satyriasis occurs and this leads to one of its main uses in veterinary practice – to control excessive sexual activity. The uterine action should not be overlooked.

### UVA URSI. Bearberry. N.O. Ericaceae.

The Ø is prepared from dried leaves and fruit.

The active principles are associated with disturbances of the urinary system. Cystitis commonly occurs and the urine may contain blood, pus and mucus. Kidney involvement is usually confined to the pelvis causing a purulent inflammation. This is one of the main remedies used in the treatment of cystitis and pyelonephritis.

### VARIOLINUM.

This is the nosode of smallpox and in veterinary practice has given good results in the control and treatment of the different poxes affecting cattle and goats.

### VERATRUM ALBUM. White Hellebore. N.O. Liliaceae.

The Ø is prepared from root stocks.

A picture of collapse is presented by the action of this plant. Extremities become cold and signs of cyanosis appear. Purging occurs, the watery diarrhoea being accompanied by exhaustion. The body surface quickly becomes cold and the stools are greenish. Signs of abdominal pain precede the onset of diarrhoea.

## VIBURNUM OPULIS, Water Elder. Cranberry.
### N.O. Caprifoliaceae.
The Ø is prepared from the fresh bark.

Muscular cramps are associated with the action of this plant. The female genital system is markedly affected, chiefly the uterus, producing a tendency to abortion in the first quarter of pregnancy, sterility being a common sequel. It is principally used in the treatment of animals with a history of repeated miscarriages.

## VIPERA. Common Viper.
Potencies are prepared from diluted venom.

This poison causes paresis of the hind limbs with a tendency to paralysis. Symptoms extend upwards. Skin and subcutaneous tissues become swollen after a bite, with livid tongue and swollen lips developing. Disturbances of liver function produce a jaundice of visible mucous membranes. Inflammation of veins occurs with attendant oedema. Oedematous states arising from venous congestion provide conditions suitable for its use and it should be remembered as a possibly useful remedy in liver dysfunction.

## ZINCUM METALLICUM. Zinc. The Metal.
Potencies are prepared from trituration with subsequent dilution in alcohol.

This element produces a state of anaemia with a decrease in the number of red cells. There is a tendency to fall towards the left side with weakness and trembling of muscles. It is a useful remedy in suppressed feverish states accompanied by anaemia and may prove useful in brain conditions showing typical symptoms.

# NOSODES AND ORAL VACCINES

Reference to nosodes and oral vaccines has already been made in the Introduction to this book, and it is only necessary to add that all disease products are rendered innocuous after the third centesimal potency which is equivalent to a strength or dilution of 1/1,000,000. They are used in the 30c potency.

## BACILLINUM.

This remedy is prepared from tuberculous material. It has a limited use in goat keeping, but it is extremely useful in the treatment of ringworm and similar sklin diseases.

## CARCINOSIN.

The Nosode of Carcinoma.

This little used remedy in goat keeping can be helpful in cases of glandular enlargements accompanied by feverish states.

## E COLI. *Nosode and Oral Vaccine.*

Prepared from various strains of E. Coli. It has been found in practice that the strain which has given the most consistent results is the one which was prepared originally from a human source. Both treatment and prevention of coli-bacillosis come within its range and also the specific form of mastitis associated with E. Coli infection.

## FOLLICULINUM.

The nosode prepared from the corpus luteum is used chiefly in the treatment of various ovarian and allied conditions.

## OOPHORINUM.

This is the actual ovarian hormone. Ovarian troubles come within its sphere of action, e.g. sterility dependent on ovarian dysfunction. It has also been used in some forms of skin disorder thought to be associated with hormone imbalance.

## PSORINUM. *Scabies Vesicle.*

This is a valuable skin remedy. It is not often called for in goat practice, but should be kept in mind as a possibly useful addition to the more commonly used remedies. Ringworm may respond, as well as other conditions attended by dry coat and great itching.

## PYROGENIUM. *Pyrogen.*

This nosode is prepared from decaying animal protein. Despite its origin it is an extremely valuable remedy in the treatment of septicaemic or toxaemic states where vital reserves are low. One of the main indications for its use is illness attended by a high temperature alternating with a weak thready pulse, or alternatively a low temperature with a firm pulse. All discharges and septic states are extremely offensive. It could have a vital part to play in puerperal feverish conditions, and has been used in retained afterbirth after abortions.

### SALMONELLA. *Nosode and Oral Vaccine.*
Prepared from the common Salmonella organisms associated with this disease and used both prophylactically and therapeutically.

### STREPTOCOCCUS. *Nosode an d Oral Vaccine.*
Prepared from strains of haemolytic streptococci. It is used in various infections associated with these bacteria.

### SYCOTIC CO. *One of the Bowel Nosodes.*
This is one of a group of nosodes prepared from the non-lactose fermenting bacilli found in the large intestine. Each one is related to certain homoeopathic remedies and used mainly in conjunction with them. They are also used by themselves. Sycotic Co. has been used successfully in intestinal conditions producing catarrhal inflammation on mucous membranes.

### TUBERCULINUM AVIARE.
Avian sources provide the material for this nosode.

This nosode may prove useful in the treatment of some forms of pneumonia, along with indicated remedies. Chronic conditions are the most likely to benefit.

# *Index*

Abies Canadensis 107
  for:
    indigestion 6
abortion
  disease–induced 100
  enzootic (chlamydiosis) 82
  hormone imbalance–induced 96
  prevention by Viburnum Opulis
    use 99
abortus 100
Abrotanum 107
abscess 37–8
Absinthum 107
acetonaemia (ketosis) 52–3
Acidum Nitricum
  for:
    contagious ophthalmia 85
    Johne's disease 68
    orf 76
    stomatitis 1–2
    warts on teats 43
Acidum Salicylicum 107–8
  for:
    CAE 75
Aconitum napellus 108
  for:
    acetonaemia 53
    acidosis 55
    acute nephritis 29
    catarrhal rhinitis 12
    coccidiosis 80
    coli-bacillosis 63
    contagious ophthalmia 85
    encephalitis 27
    enteritis 7
    heat stress 43
    joint ill 65
    laminitis 51
    laryngitis 15
    lung haemorrhage 18
    mastitis 47
    meningitis 25
    metritis 102–3

navel ill 65
nose bleed 12
parotitis 3
peritonitis 8
pharyngitis 4
salmonellosis 72
snake bite 90
stomatitis 1
tetanus 62
tracheitis 16
Actaea Racemosa (Cimicifuga
  Racemosa) 108
Adonis Vernalis 108
Aesculus Hippocastanum 108–9
  for:
    lung oedema 18
    pharyngitis 4
Agaricus Muscarius 109
  for:
    CAE 75
    cerebral oedema 26
    louping ill 72–3
    poisoning by lead 92
Agnus Castus 109
  for:
    milk deficiency 48
Aletris Farinosa 109
  for:
    endocrine dysfunction 97
Allium Cepa 109–10
  for:
    catarrhal rhinitis 13
    Johne's disease 68
Alumen 110
  for:
    pharyngitis 4
Ammonium Carbonicum 110
  for:
    lung congestion 17
    lung oedema 18
    parasitic bronchitis 86
    prunus poisoning 92
    pulmonary emphysema 22

Ammonium Causticum 110
for:
  enzootic pneumonia 70
  lung congestion 17
  lung oedema 18
Angustura Vera 111
Anthracinum 111
Antimonium Arsenicosum 111
for:
  enzootic pneumonia 69–70
  lung congestion 17
  lung oedema 18
  mycoplasma infection 83
  parasitic bronchitis 86
  pulmonary emphysema 22
Antimonium Crudum 111
for:
  bloat 9
  goat pox 42
Antimonium Tartaricum 111–12
for:
  lung congestion 17
  lung oedema 18
  maedi visna 75
  parasitic bronchitis 86
  pneumonia 20
Apis Mellifica 112
for:
  acute nephritis 29
  bloat 9
  cerebral oedema 26
  cloud burst/pseudo pregnancy 101
  cystic ovaries 98
  lung congestion 17
  lung oedema 18
  mastitis 47
  meningitis 26
  pleurisy 22
  ranula 2
Apocynum Cannabinum 112
Apomorphinum 112
Argentum Nitricum 113
for:
  contagious ophthalmia 85
  Q fever 84
Arnica Montana 113
for:
  blood in milk 48
  bruise injury 91
  cerebral oedema 26
  haemorrhage 89–90
  lung haemorrhage 19
  mastitis 47
  nose bleed 11

  post-partum haemorrhage 101
  pregnancy 100
Arsenicum album 113
for:
  acute nephritis 29
  catarrhal rhinitis 12
  coccidiosis 80
  eczema 35
  enteritis 7
  enterotoxaemia 61
  photosensitisation 37
  pulmonary emphysema 22–3
  salmonellosis 72
Arsenicum iodatum 113–14
for:
  parasitic bronchitis 86–7
  pleurisy 22
Asafoetida 114
for:
  milk deficiency 49
Atropinum 114

Bacillinum nosode 114, 158
for:
  ringworm 41
Bacteria-induced disease 61–72
Baptisia Tinctora 114
Baryta Carbonica 114–15
for:
  parotitis 3
Baryta Muriatica 115
behaviour observation xiii
Belladonna 115
for:
  encephalitis 27
  heat stress 43
  hypocalcaemia 52
  hypomagnesaemia 54
  laminitis 51
  mastitis 47
  meningitis 25
  metritis 103
  nose bleed 11
  parotitis 3
  peritonitis 8
  pharyngitis 4
  poisoning by lead/prunus 92
  stomatitis 2
Bellis Perennis 115
for:
  mastitis 47
  pregnancy 100
Benzoicum Acidum 115–16
for:
  joint ill 65

Benzoicum Acidum
for: – continued
navel ill 65
pyelonephritis 31
Berberis Vulgaris 116
for:
acute nephritis 29
bladder stones 33
jaundice 10
liver function 10
Beryllium 116
for:
enzootic pneumonia 69
pneumonia 20
bladder
inflammation 32
stones (urinary calculi) 33
bloat 8–9; *see also* indigestion
blowfly 87
blue tongue 76
Borax 116
for:
gingivitis 5
stomatitis 1
Bothrops Lanceolatus 117
for:
haemorrhage 90
snake bite 91
Bromium 117
Broncho-pneumonia 68
Brucella sp. infection, abortion
induced by 100
Bryonia Alba 117
for:
degenerative joint disease 60
enzootic pneumonia 69
joint ill 65
mastitis 47
mycoplasma infection 83
navel ill 65
parotitis 3
peritonitis 8
pleurisy 21–2
pneumonia 20
pulmonary emphysema 22
tracheitis 16
Bufo 117–18

Cactus Grandiflorus 118
CAE (caprine arthritis encephalitis)
73–5
Calcarea Carbonica 118
for warts on teats 42–3
Calcarea Fluorica 118
for:
caseous lymphadenitis 70

laminitis 51
mastitis 48
mycoplasma infection 83
parotitis 3
seedy toe 67
Calcarea Iodata 118–19
Calcarea Phosphorica 119
for:
early abortion 96
frequent return to service 99
hypocalcaemia 52
kid rearing 105
oestrus cycle initiation 97
osteodystrophia fibrosa 56–7
rickets 59
Calc. Renalis Phosph. 119
Calc. Renalis Uric. 119
Calcium Carbonate, for
degenerative joint disease 60
calcium deficiency 51–2
calcium/phosphorus imbalance
56, 59
Calendula Officinalis 119
Calendula/Hypericum lotion *see*
Hypercal
Calendula/Hypericum/Cineraria
eye lotion 85
Calici Virus nosode 119
Camphora 119–20
for coli-bacillosis 64
Cannabis Sativa 120
for mycoplasma infection 83
Cantharis 120
for:
cystitis 32
peritonitis 8
caprine arthritis encephalitis (CAE)
73–5
Carbo Vegetabilis 120
for:
acidosis 55
bloat 9
coli-bacillosis 64
indigestion 6
poisoning by prunus 92
suppurative pneumonia 211
Carcinosin 158
Carduus Marianus 121
for ragwort poisoning 92
caseous lymphadenitis 70–1
control 71
catarrh
chronic nasal (chronic rhinitis)
13–14

Caulophyllum 121
for:
  chlamydiosis (enzootic abortion)
    82
  cloud burst/pseudo pregnancy
    prevention 101
  pregnancy 99–100
Causticum 121
for:
  cystitis 32
  warts on teats 43
Causticum/Thuja ointment 43
cellulitis 38
Ceonothus Americanus 121–2
cerebral oedema 26–7
Chelidonium 122
for:
  jaundice 9–10
  liver function 10
  photosensitisation 37
  poisoning by ragwort 92
Chenopodium, for worming 93
Chimaphilla Umbellata 122
  for pyelonephritis 32
China *see* Cinchona Officinalis
Chininum Sulphuricum 122
Chionanthus Virginia 122–3
for:
  jaundice 10
  liver function 10
  ragwort poisoning 92
Chlamydia sp. infection
  abortion induced by 100
  prevention by nosode use 123
*Chlamydia psittaci* 82
chlamydiosis (enzootic abortion) 82
chorioptic (leg) mange 39
Cicuta Virosa 123
for:
  acetonaemia 53
  CAE 74
  cerebral oedema 26
  listeriosis 79
  louping ill 73
  meningitis 25
  poisoning by lead 92
Cinchona Officinalis (China) 123
for:
  coccidiosis 80
  coli-bacillosis 64
  kale (rape poisoning) 92
Cineraria Maritima 123
  Cineraria/Hypericum/Calendula
  eye lotion 85

Cinnabaris 124
Circling disease (listeriosis) 79–80
*Clostridium tetani* 62
cobalt deficiency (pine) 57–8
Cobaltum 124
  for cobalt deficiency 58
Cobaltum Chloride 124
  for cobalt deficiency 58
Cobra venom (Naja Tripudians) 90,
  142–3
coccidiosis 80–1
Cocculus 124
Coccus Cacti 124
Colchicum Autumnale 124–5
for:
  acidosis 55
  bloat 9
  indigestion 6
  rhododendron poisoning 91
coli-bacillosis (white/dietary scour)
  63–4
Colocynthis 125
for:
  cystic ovaries 98
  cystitis 32–3
  enteritis 7
  rhododendron poisoning 91
Condurango 125
Conium Maculatum 125
for:
  CAE 74
  hypocalcaemia 52
  louping ill 73
  swayback (enzootic ataxia) 57
contagious agalactica 83
contagious ophthalmia (New Forest
  disease) 84–5
contagious pleuro-pneumonia 83
contagious pustular dermatitis (orf)
  76–7
Copaiva 126
for:
  acute nephritis 30
  cystitis 32
  pyelonephritis 31
corpus luteum, persistent 98–9
Convallaria Majalis 126
Cortisone 126
*Corynebacterium ovis* 70
  nosode 71
coryza (catarrhal rhinitis) 12–13
*Coxilla burnetti* 84
Crataegus 126

Crotalus Horridus 126–7
  for:
    blood in milk 48
    haemorrhage 90
    nose bleed 12
    poisoning by kale (rape) 92
    post-partum haemorrhage 101
    snake bite 91
Croton Tiglium 127
  for enteritis 7
Cryptococcus nosode 127
Cubeba Officinalis (Cu Bebs) 127
  for cystitis 32
Cuprum Aceticum 127
  for:
    goat pox 42
    hypomagnesaemia 54
Cuprum Metallicum 127–8
  for:
    encephalitis 27
    swayback prevention 57
    vitamin E deficiency 60
Curare 128
  for:
    tetanus 62
    vitamin E deficiency 60
cystic ovaries 98
cystitis 32–3

Damiana 128
demodectic mange 39, 40
dermatitis, contagious pustular (orf)
  76–7
diet, high concentrate/associated
  problems
    acidosis 54
    bladder stones 33
dietary scour (coli-bacillosis; white
  scour) 63–4
Digitalis Purpurea 128
drinking water 33
Drosera Rotundifolia 128
  for:
    enzootic pneumonia 69
    pneumonia 20
    pulmonary emphysema 22
    tracheitis 16
Dulcamara 128–9
  for:
    catarrhal rhinitis 13
    coli-bacillosis 64
    tracheitis 16

Echinacea Augustifolia 129
  for:

eczema 36
  metritis 103
eczema 35–6
Eel Serum 129
  for acute nephritis 30
Eimeria sp. 80
encephalitis 27
encephalomalacia 26
endocrine dysfunction 96–7
  frequent return to service due to
    99
enteritis 7–8
enterotoxaemia 61
enzootic ataxia (swayback) 57
enzootic pneumonia (pasteurellosis)
  68–70
*Epigea repens* 120
epistaxis (nose bleed) 11–12
*Escherichia coli*
  intestinal disturbance induced by
    63
  nosode/oral vaccine (*E. coli*) 129,
    158
      for coli-bacillosis 64
Euphrasia Officinalis 129–30
eye lotion 85

facial urticaria 37
F.V.R. (feline viral rhinotracheitis)
  nosode 130
Ferrum Phosphoricum 130
  for:
    catarrhal rhinitis 12
    enzootic pneumonia 69
    lung congestion 17
    maedi visna 75–6
    mycoplasma infection 83
    pneumonia 20
    sinusitis 14
Ficus Religiosa 130
  for:
    blood in milk 48
    lung haemorrhage 19
    nose bleed 12
    post-partum haemorrhage 101
first-aid 89–92
Flor de Piedra (*also known as*
  Lophophytum) 131
  for:
    acetonaemia 53
    iodine deficiency 58–9
Fluoricum Acidum 131
Folliculinum nosode 131, 158
  for:
    endocrine dysfunction 97

Folliculinum nosode
  for: – continued
    persistent corpus luteum 98
foot rot 65–6
Formica 13
*Fusiformis nodosus* 65

Gaertner-Bach 131
  for Johne's disease 68
Galega Officinalis 131–2
  for excess mik secretion 49
Gelsemium Sempervirens 132
  for hypomagnesaemia 54
gingivitis 5–6
Glonoinum 132
goat pox 40–2
Granatum, for worming 93
Graphites 132
  for:
    eczema 36
    mange 40
grass tetany (hypomagnesaemia)
  53–4
Green Mussel, for CAE 75
gums, inflammation of (gingivitis)
  5–6
Gunpowder 132
  for:
    abscess 38
    caseous lymphadenitis 70–1

haemoglobinuria 67
haemorrhage 89–90
  lung 19
  post-partum 101–2
Hamamelis Virginica 133
  for:
    nose bleed 12
    post-partum haemorrhage 101
heat stress 43
Hecla Lava 133
  for degenerative joint disease 60
Helleborus Niger 133
Hepar Sulphuris Calcareum 133–4
  for:
    abscess 38
    eczema 36
    foot rot 66
    mange 40
    mastitis 48
    purulent nephritis 30–1
    pyelonephritis 31
    seedy toe 67
    sinusitis 14
    suppurative pneumonia 21

high concentrate diet/associated
  problems of:
    acidosis 54
    bladder stones 33
Hippozaeninum 134
homoeopathy, description xiii; *see
  also* remedy
Hydrangea Arborescens 134
  for bladder stones 33
Hydrastis Canadensis 134
  for:
    catarrhal rhinitis 13
    chronic rhinitis 13
Hydrocotyle Asiatica 134
hydrogen peroxide, Hypercal
  combined with 38
Hyoscyamus Niger 134–5
Hypercal lotion
  for:
    abscess 38
    external parasites 87
    goat pox 42
    orf 77
    seedy toe 67
    teat injury 48–9
    wound/laceration 89
*Hypericum perforatum* (St John's
  Wort), ingestion 36
Hypericum Perforatum 135
  for:
    photosensitisation 37
    tetanus 62
    wound/laceration 89
Hypericum/Calendula lotion *see*
  Hypercal lotion
Hypericum/Calendula/Cineraria
  eye lotion 85
hypocalcaemia (milk fever) 51–2
hypomagnesaemia (grass tetany)
  53–4
Hyoscyamus, for encephalitis 27

indigestion
  acute 6–7
  bloat 9
infertility 95–103
  causes 96–7
iodine deficiency 58–9
Iodum 135
  for:
    iodine deficiency 58
    oestrus cycle initiation 97
Ipecacuanha 135
  for:
    blood in milk 48

Ipecacuanha
 for: – continued
  coccidiosis 80–1
  haemorrhage 90
  lung haemorrhage 19
  post-partum haemorrhage 101
Iris Versicolour 136
*Ixodes ricinus* 72

jaundice 9–10
Johne's disease 67–8
joint disease, degenerative 60
joint ill 64–5

kale (rape) poisoning 91–2
Kali Arsenicum 136
 for:
  mange 40
  ringworm 41
Kali Bichromicum 136
 for:
  chronic rhinitis 13
  goat pox 42
  sinusitis 14
Kali Carbonicum 136
 for pleurisy 22
Kali Chloricum 136
Kali Hydriodicum 136–7
Kali Iod., for contagious
ophthalmia 85
Kamala, for worming 93
keratitis 83
Ketosis (acetonaemia) 52–3
kid
 rearing 105
 weak 82
kidney
 abscess (purulent nephritis) 30–1
 inflammation (acute nephritis)
  29–30
knee joint affection 64–5
Kreosotum 137
 for root rot 66

Labour, difficult, metritis following
 102–3
laceration 89
Lachesis 137
 for:
  haemorrhage 90
  laryngitis 15
  metritis 103
  pharyngitis 4
  snake bite 90–1
laminitis 51

laryngitis 15–16
Lathyrus Sativus 137
 for swayback 57
lead poisoning 92
Ledum Palustre 137–8
 for:
  joint ill 65
  mycoplasma infection 83
  navel ill 65
  snake bite 91
  tetanus 62
  wound/laceration 89
leg mange (chorioptic mange) 39
Lemna Minor 138
leptospirosis 67
lice 87
'likes be cured by likes, let' xiv
Lilium Tigrinum 138
listeria nosode 80
listeriosis (Circling disease) 79–80
  abortion induced by 100
Lithium Carbonicum 138
liver dysfunction 10
Lobelia Inflata 138
 for pulmonary emphysema 22
Lophophytum *see* Flor de Piedra
louping ill 72–3
lung
 congestion 16–17
 haemorrhage 18–19
 oedema 17–18
lungworm disease (parasitic
 bronchitis) 86–7
Lycoplus Virginicus 139
Lycopodium Clavatum 139
 for:
  acetonaemia 53
  bladder stones 33
  bloat 9
  ingestion 6
  jaundice 10
  liver function 10
  maedi visna 75–6
  mycoplasma infection 83
  pneumonia 20
  poisoning by ragwort 92
  pregnancy toxaemia 56

maedi visna 75
Magnesia Phosphorica 139
 for:
  hypocalcaemia 52
  hypomagnesaemia 54
  meningitis 26
  pregnancy toxaemia 56

Magnesia Phosphorica
 for: – continued
  vitamin E deficiency 60
Malandrinum 139–40
 for mange 40
male goat, bladder stones in 33
mange 39–40
mastitis 45–8
 acute 45
 chronic 45–6
 homoeopathic control 46
 treatment 47–8
mating, refusal to participate in 96
Medusa 140
 for excess milk secretion 49
Melilotus 140
 for:
  blood in milk 48
  haemorrhage 90
  lung haemorrhage 19
  nose bleed 11
  post-partum haemorrhage 101
Melitensis 100
meningitis 25–6
meningo-encephalitis 72
mental symptom xiii
Mercurius *see* Mercurius Solubis
Mercurius Corrosivus 140
 for:
  catarrhal rhinitis 13
  coccidiosis 81
  eczema 36
  enteritis 7
  gingivitis 5
  pyelonephritis 31
  laryngitis 15
  pharyngitis 4
Mercurius Dulcis 141
 for ranula 2
Mercurius Iodatus Flavus 141
 for gingivitis 5
Mercurius Iodatus Ruber 141
 for gingivitis 5
Mercurius Solubis (Mercurius) 140
 for:
  caseous lymphadenitis 71
  chronic rhinitis 13–14
  gingivitis 5
  Q fever 84
  sinusitis 14
  stomatitis 1
metritis, puerperal 102–3
 acute 102
milk
 blood in 48

deficiency 49
excess secretion 49
milk fever (hypocalcaemia) 51–2
Millefolium 141
 for:
  blood in milk 48
  haemorrhage 90
  lung haemorrhage 19
  nose bleed 11
  post-partum haemorrhage 101
Mineral Extract 141–2
Mixed Grasses 142
Morgan-Bach 142
 for eczema 35
mouth inflammation (stomatitis)
 1–2
multiple arthritis infection 83
Murex Purpurea 142
 for cystic ovaries 98
Muriatic Acid 142
*Myocbacterium Johnei* 68
mycoplasma infection 82–4
 abortion induced by 100
 control 83–4
Myristica Sebifera 142
 for seedy toe 67

Naja Tripudians (Cobra venom) 90,
 142–3
Natrum Muriaticum 143
 for cystic ovaries 98
Natrum Sulphoricum 143
navel ill 64–5
nephritis
 acute 29–30
 purulent (kidney abscess) 30–1
New Forest disease (contagious
 ophthalmia) 84–5
Nitricum Acidum 143
Norwegian Dairy 36
nose bleed (epistaxis) 11–12
nosodes xvi, 157–9
Nux Vomica 143–4
 for:
  acetonaemia 53
  acidosis 55
  indigestion 6
  rhododendron poisoning 91

Ocimum Canum 144
 for pyelonephritis 31–2
oestrus cycle
 irregularities 96–100
 stages 95–6, 97
  anoestrus 96, 97

oestrus cycle
  stages: – continued
    dioestrus 95
    metoestrus 95
    oestrus 95
    pro-oestrus 95
oocyst 80
Oopherinum nosode 158
  for:
    cloud burst/pseudo pregnancy
      101
    cystic ovaries 98
    frequent return to service 99
opisthotonus 27
Opium 144
oral vaccine xvi, 157–9
orf (contagious pustular dermatitis)
  76–7
osteodystrophia fibrosa 56–7
Ovarium 144
ovulation failure 99

Palladium 144
  for:
    cloud burst/pseudo pregnancy
      prevention 101
Pancreas 144
parasites, external 87
parasitic bronchitis (lungworm
  disease) 86–7
Pareira 144–5
Parotidinum 145
  for parotitis 3–4
parotitis 2–4
parturition
  anoestrus following 97
  problems following 101–3
Pasteurella nosode 145
pasteurellosis (enzootic pneumonia)
  19, 68–70
peritonitis 8–9
persistent corpus luteum 98–9
Petroleum 145
pharyngitis 4–5
Phosphoricum Acidum 145
  for rickets 59
Phosphorus 145
  for:
    caseous lymphadenitis 71
    enzootic pneumonia
      (pasteurellosis) 69
    haemorrhage 90
    jaundice 10
    liver function 10
    lung haemorrhage 19

  maedi visna 75
  mycoplasma infection 83
  nose bleed 12
  pneumonia 20
  poisoning by ragwort 92
  post-partum haemorrhage 102
  pregnancy toxaemia 56
  Q fever 84
Phosphorus/calcium imbalance 56,
  59
photosensitisation 36–7
Phytolacca Decandra 146
  for:
    laryngitis 15
    mastitis 47
    parotitis 3
pine (cobalt deficiency) 57–8
pituitrin injection, replacement for
  100
placenta
  retained 102
    puerperal metritis following
      102–3
Platina
  for:
    cloud burst/pseudo pregnancy
      101
    cystic ovaries 98
    endocrine dysfunction 97
pleurisy 21–2
Plumbum Metallicum 146
  for:
    encephalitis 27
    meningitis 26
    poisoning by lead 92
pneumonia 19–20
  broncho-pneumonia 19
  pasteurella (enzootic pneumonia)
    19, 68–70
  suppurative (pulmonary abscess)
    21
Podophyllum 146
poisoning 91–2
post-partum
  complications 101–3
  use of:
    Arnica Montana 100
    Bellis Perennis 100
potentisation xiv
pregnancy 99–100
  associated problems 100–1
  cloud burst 100–1
  post-partum complications 101–3
  pseudo 100–1
pregnancy toxaemia 55–6

prunus poisoning 92
Pseudomonas 146
Psorinum nosode 146–7, 158
  for mange 40
psoroptic mange 39
Ptelea 147
puerperal metritis 102–3
  acute 102
pulmonary abscess (suppurative
  pneumonia) 21
pulmonary emphysema 22–3
Pulsatilla 147
  for:
    early abortion 96
    catarrhal rhinitis 13
    cloud burst/pseudo pregnancy
      101
    coli-bacillosis 63–4
    endocrine dysfunction 97
    frequent return to service 99
    oestrus cycle initiation 97
    parotitis 3
    persistent corpus luteum 98–9
    retained placenta 102
pyelonephritis 31–2
Pyrogenium nosode 147, 158–9
  for:
    coli-bacillosis 64
    enterotoxaemia 61
    metritis 103
    peritonitis 7–8
    purulent nephritis 30
    Q fever 84
    retained placenta 102
    salmonellosis 72

Q fever 84

ragwort poisoning 92
ranula 2
Ranunculus Bulbosus 147
  for goat pox 42
rape (kale) poisoning 91–2
remedy
  administration xv
  care xv–xvi
  potency xv
  preparation (potentisation) xiv–xv
  *see also* homoeopathy, description
reproduction *see* oestrus cycle
rescue remedy 147–8
retrovirus group 74
Rheum 148
  for enteritis 7
rhinitis 12

catarrhal (coryza) 12–13
chronic (chronic nasal catarrh)
  13–14
Rhododendron 148
rhododendron poisoning 91
Rhus Toxicodendron 148
  for:
    CAE 74–5
    orf (contagious pustular
      dermatitis) 77
    parotitis 3
    peritonitis 8
    pharyngitis 5
    photosensitisation 37
    rhododendron poisoning 91
rickets 59
ringworm 40–1
Rumex Crispus 148
Ruta Graveolens 148–9
  for:
    joint ill 65
    mycoplasma 83
    navel ill 65

Saanen 36
Sabina 149
  for:
    chlamydiosis (enzootic abortion)
      82
    metritis 103
    retained placenta 102
St John's Wort (*Hypericum
  perforatum*), ingestion 36
Salmonella
  nosode 72, 159
  oral vaccine 159
salmonellosis 71–2
  abortion induced by 100
  prevention 72
Sanguinaria 149
  for laryngitis 15
sarcoptic mange 39
scrapie 81
Secale Cornutum 149
  for:
    chlamydiosis (enzootic abortion)
      82
    metritis 103
    post-partum haemorrhage 101
seedy toe 66–7
Selenium deficiency (*also known as*
  vitamin E deficiency) 59–60
Sepia Officinalis 149–50
  for:
    chlamydiosis (enzootic abortion) 82

Sepia Officinalis
 for: – continued
  cloud burst/pseudo pregnancy
   101
  endocrine dysfunction 96–7
  frequent return to service 99
  persistent corpus luteum 99
  refusal to mate 96
  retained placenta 102
service, frequent return to 99
sheep scab, psoroptic mange
 compared with 39
Silicea 150
 for:
  abscess 38
  caseous lymphadenitis 70
  chronic rhinitis 14
  contagious ophthalmia 85
  foot rot 66
  mastitis 48
  mycoplasma infection 83
  purulent nephritis 30
  pyelonephritis 31
  seedy toe 67
  sinusitis 14
  suppurative pneumonia 21
sinusitis 14
snake bite 90–1
snake venom-based remedy 90
Solidago Virga 150
Spigella 150
Spongia Tosta 150–1
 for laryngitis 15
Squilla Maritima 151
S.S.C., for mastitis 47–8
Staphisagria 151
Staphylococcus nosode 151
 for abscess 38
*Staphylococcus aureus* 46, 151
*Staphylococcus pyogenes* 46
stillbirth 82
Stramonium 151
 for:
  CAE 74
  cerebral oedema 26
  encephalitis 27
  listeriosis 79
  louping ill 73
  poisoning by lead 92
Streptococcus nosode/oral vaccine
 151, 159
 for:
  abscess 38
  joint ill 65
  navel ill 65

*Streptococcus agalactiae* 46
*Streptococcus dysgalactiae* 46
*Streptococcus pyogenes* 46
stomatitis 1–2
Strophanthus 151–2
Strychinum 152
 for:
  cerebral oedema 27
  tetanus 62
Sulfonal 152
 for:
  listeriosis 79
  poisoning by lead 92
  swayback (enzootic ataxia) 57
  eczema 35
  mange 40
  photosensitisation 37
swayback (enzootic ataxia) 57
Sycotic Co. nosode 159
 for coccidiosis 81
Symphytum 152–3
Syzygium 153

Tabacum 153
Tarentula Cubensis 153
 for:
  abscess 38
  caseous lymphadenitis 71
Tarentula Hispanica 153
teats
 injury to 48–9
 warts on 42–3
Tellurium 153
 for ringworm 41
Terebinthinae 154
 for acute nephritis 30
Testosterone 154
tetanus/tetanus nosode 62–3
Thallium Acetas 154
Thlaspi Bursa Pastoralis 154
 for bladder stones 33
throat inflammation (pharyngitis) 4
Thuja Occidentalis 154–5
 Thuja/Causticum ointment 43
Thyroidium 155
tick 87
 louping ill transmission by 72
tongue, swelling beneath 2
toxoplasma infection, abortion
 induced by 100
toxoplasmosis 84
*Toxoplasmosis gondii* 84
tracheitis 16
Trichophyton nosode, for
 ringworm 41

*Trichophyton verrucosum* 40
Trinitrotoluene 155
Tuberculinum Aviare nosode 159
  for:
    enzootic pneumonia
      (pasteurellosis) 69
    pneumonia 20
Tuberculinum Bovinum nosode
  155
  for mastitis 48
twins/associated risks 55

Uranium Nitricum 155
Urtica Urens 155–6
  for:
    excess milk secretion 49
    facial urticaria 37
    milk deficiency 49
urticaria, facial 37
urinary calculi (bladder stones) 33
Ustillago Maydis 156
uterine endometrium
  hyperplasia of 98
  inflammation (puerperal metritis)
    102–3
Uva Ursi 156
  for acute nephritis 30

vaccination procedure xvi–xvii
vaccine, oral xvi, 157–9
Variolinum 156
  for goat pox/goat pox prevention
    42
Veratrum Album 156
  for coccidiosis 81
  coli-bacillosis 63
  salmonellosis 72
Viburnum Opulis 157
  for:
    early abortion 96
    pregnancy/abortion prevention
      99
Vipera 157
  for:
    haemorrhage 90
    nose bleed 12
    snake bite 91
virus-induced disease 72–77
vitamins
  B12
    production 57
    supplements 58
  D deficiency 59
  E deficiency (*also known as*
    selenium deficiency) 59–60

warts on teats 42–3
white scour (coli-bacillosis; dietary
  scour) 63–4
windpipe inflammation 16
worming 93
wound 89

Zincum Metallicum 157
  for meningitis 25–6